COLOUR
ATLAS
OF
OPHTHALMOLOGY

IOP Publishing Limited

Published under the Wright imprint by

IOP Publishing Limited
Techno House, Redcliffe Way
Bristol BS1 6NX England

1st English Edition	—	1979
Malay Edition	—	1981
Spanish Edition	—	1981
English Edition (Reprint)	—	1982
Italian Edition	—	1984
Chinese Edition	—	1984
English Edition (Reprint)	—	1984
English Edition (Paperback)	—	1985
French Edition	—	1985
Finnish Edition	—	1987
English Edition (Second)	—	1987
English Edition (Paperback)	—	1987

British Library Cataloguing in Publication Data
Lim, Arthur Siew Ming
Colour Atlas Of Ophthalmology — 2nd ed
1. Ophthalmology
I. Title II. Constable, Ian J
617.7 RE46
ISBN 0-7236-0947-0

Printed in Singapore
by Tien Wah Press (Pte) Ltd, 977, Bukit Timah Road, Singapore 2158

COLOUR
ATLAS
OF
OPHTHALMOLOGY

with 199 illustrations, 187 in colour

ARTHUR LIM SIEW MING
MBBS AM FRACS FRACO FRCS DO

Chief, Department of Ophthalmology
National University Hospital and
Visiting Consultant, Ministry of Health
Republic of Singapore

Visiting Professor
Sun Yat-Sen University of Medical Sciences and
Tianjin Medical College and
Honorary Visiting Professor
Beijing Medical University
People's Republic of China

IAN J CONSTABLE
MBBS FRCSE FRACS FRACO

Lion's Professor of Ophthalmology
University of Western Australia

Director
Lions Eye Institute, Perth, Australia

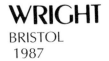

WRIGHT
BRISTOL
1987

THE AUTHORS

Dr Arthur S M Lim is the Chief of the Department of Ophthalmology, National University Hospital and the Visiting Consultant in ophthalmology to the Ministry of Health of the Republic of Singapore. He is also the Visiting Professor to the Sun Yat-sen University of Medical Sciences, the People's Republic of China; and the Honorary Visiting Professor, Beijing Medical University and the Visiting Professor to the Tianjin Medical College, the People's Republic of China. Dr. Lim is External Examiner, Master of Surgery (Ophthalmology), Universiti Kebangsaan Malaysia.

Dr Lim is the President of the Asia Pacific Academy of Ophthalmology and the President of the 26th International Congress of Ophthalmology which will be held in Singapore in 1990. He is a recipient of the Jose Rizal Medal for excellence in ophthalmology in the Asia Pacific region, the highest award of the Asia Pacific Academy of Ophthalmology. He is a member of the Academia Ophthalmologica Internationalis.

Dr Lim has written seven books. To date, Dr Lim has published 170 scientific papers and is on the editorial boards of eight international scientific journals.

Professor Ian Constable is a diplomate of the American Board of Ophthalmologists and Fellow of the Royal College of Surgeons, Edinburgh, Royal Australasian College of Surgeons and the Royal Australian College of Ophthalmologists. He is currently Lions Professor of Ophthalmology, University of Western Australia and Director of the Lions Eye Institute, Perth.

He was formerly an Associate Scientist at the Retina Foundation, Boston, Assistant Surgeon at the Massachusetts Eye and Ear Infirmary, and an Instructor in Ophthalmology at Harvard Medical School, Boston, USA.

He has published extensively on the retina and vitreous and is co-author with Dr Arthur S M Lim of the textbook Laser: Its Clinical Uses in Eye Diseases.

PREFACE

In the last decade, advances in colour technology have made it possible to reproduce high quality colour photographs at a reasonable cost. This has been of tremendous value in the teaching of ophthalmology, as the vividness of the colour photographs adds clarity to the written word.

It is our hope that this colour atlas will be a useful guide not only to general practitioners, but to other non-ophthalmologists as well — the physicians, surgeons, nurses, students and all those paramedical personnel who have to deal with common eye diseases. Some practical geographical and racial differences have been included to emphasize the growing importance of the different disease patterns in different countries.

This volume is kept small and handy and the text brief, in order that busy practitioners, students and others who may refer to it, will not be unnecessarily burdened with theories which are controversial, or with eye diseases of little practical importance.

ASM Lim
IJ Constable

PREFACE TO SECOND EDITION

Eight years have passed since the publication of the First Edition of the Colour Atlas of Ophthalmology. Enthusiastic reviews from international journals, translations into six languages (Malay/Indonesian, Spanish, Italian, Chinese, French and Finnish) and requests from our readers for updated material have encouraged us to produce this new edition. Besides including new technologies such as ultrasonography and Krypton and YAG lasers which are now used in many countries, we have also inserted additional photographs and replaced old photographs with better ones. We have, however, taken pains not to increase the size of this. It is our hope that this atlas will continue to fulfil the purpose for which it was written.

ASM Lim
IJ Constable

ACKNOWLEDGEMENT

We would like to express our thanks to those who have helped to make this atlas possible.

The preparation of the manuscript was done with the invaluable help of Mrs A S M Lim, Mrs Bernice Cheng and Miss Fanny Low. Typing of the drafts and redrafts was achieved with great patience by our secretarial staff, especially Miss Helen Deady, Mrs Julie Goh and Ms Clara Cheng. The assistance of Mr Christopher Barry and Mr Patrick Goh in the preparation of illustrations is gratefully acknowledged, and we would also like to sincerely thank the Institute of Ophthalmology, London for allowing us to reproduce Figure 5.17.

The kindness of Dr Ang Beng Chong, FRACS, Dr Currie Chiang, FRCS, Dr Heng Lee Kwang, FRCS, Dr Gordon Horne, FRCPE, Dr Koh Eng Kheng, FRCGP and Dr Poh Soo Chuan, FRCPE, for reviewing the final draft of the manuscript and in helping us with their useful comments is appreciated.

Finally, a word of thanks to our publishers, P G Medical Books and Tien Wah Press (Pte) Ltd, for the publishing and printing of the Atlas.

ASM Lim
IJ Constable

CONTENTS

1

EXAMINATION

INTRODUCTION

In the assessment of a patient with eye disease, it is important to take a good history, examine the eyes with adequate illumination and test the visual function.

Recently, retinal and macular diseases have become more common as causes of severe visual loss. In these cases, a fundal examination with dilatation of the pupils in a darkened room is necessary.

HISTORY

A careful history of the patient's ocular symptoms is essential. His past history and general illnesses, such as diabetes and hypertension, frequently provide useful clues.

Myopia, squint, open-angle glaucoma and dystrophic conditions have a hereditary tendency which is revealed by an inquiry into the patient's family history. It is also useful to take note of allergies and of the medical therapy the patient is undergoing.

OCULAR SYMPTOMS

The more important symptoms include decreased visual acuity, floaters, ocular pain, headaches, itching, flashes, watering and double vision (diplopia).

Decreased visual acuity

Decreased visual acuity must always be investigated and the cause found. The cause for a sudden loss of vision could be vascular in nature such as retinal vein occlusion, retinal artery occlusion or vitreous haemorrhage. It could also be due to acute glaucoma, retinal detachment or inflammatory conditions such as acute uveitis and optic neuritis.

Gradual loss of vision is usually due to a refractive error such as myopia or presbyopia, or to degenerative conditions of which cataract is the most common. It could also be due to macular degeneration or chronic glaucoma.

Floaters

Another common ocular symptom which calls for further investigation is the appearance of floaters usually described by the patient as small, semi-translucent particles of varying shapes moving across the visual field with the movement of the eye. Single or double floaters of many months or years are common and usually harmless. But a sudden increase in floaters, especially when associated with lightning flashes and visual loss in patients with high myopia or in the elderly, suggests retinal disease, particularly retinal detachment.

Flashes

Flashes are momentary flashes of light due to stimulation of the retina and are seen in retinal tears and detachments and also in vitreous detachment. Other sensations of light may arise from migraine or lesions of the visual pathway.

Eye pain and headaches

Eye pain and headaches may be due to either ophthalmic or non-ophthalmic causes. Of the ophthalmic causes, acute glaucoma is the most important. Less frequent but just as important is iritis. Uncorrected refractive error, migraine and anxiety are common causes of headaches.

Itchy eyes

Itching around the eyes is frequently due to allergy. It may also be due to blepharitis.

Watering

In infants, watering is usually due to a blocked nasolacrimal duct. A rare but important cause of watering and irritable eyes is congenital glaucoma. Another cause is entropion of the lower lid.

In adults, watering has many causes, a common one being a blocked nasolacrimal duct. It can also occur in association with surface irritation, as in conjunctivitis, keratitis or when a foreign particle is in the eye.

Double vision (diplopia)

It is important to note whether double vision (binocular diplopia) occurs only when both eyes are opened or when one eye is occluded (monocular diplopia).

Binocular diplopia is usually due to extraocular muscle paralysis. Monocular diplopia is caused by disease in the eyeball, such as early cataract, lens dislocation or corneal opacity.

EXAMINATION

VISUAL ACUITY

The assessment of distant and near visual acuity is important as it reflects the state of the macular function (central vision). The visual acuity can be tested by asking the patient to cover one of the eyes with a cardboard or with the palm of his hand. By testing the ability of the patient to see objects such as the clock or the newspaper in his own environment, it is possible to get a gross assessment of the visual acuity as blind, grossly defective, subnormal or normal.

Distant visual acuity

It is usually necessary to record a patient's distant visual acuity more accurately with Snellen's chart. It is read at six metres, with the letters diminishing in size from above.

The patient has normal vision if he is able to read the line of letters designated as 6/6 at or near the bottom of the chart. The scale for decreasing distant visual acuity is 6/9, 6/12 (industrial vision), 6/18, 6/24, 6/36 and 6/60 (legal blindness in some countries).

If the patient is unable to read the letters, he is asked to count the examiner's fingers which are held a metre away. If his answers are correct, he has distant visual acuity of "count fingers" at a metre. If he is unable to count the fingers, the examiner should move his hand in front of the patient's eyes. The visual acuity is then said to be "hand movement". If he can see only light, visual acuity is recorded as "perception of light". If he cannot see any light, visual acuity is recorded as "no perception of light" which is total blindness.

VISUAL ACUITY TRANSCRIPTION TABLES
(Adopted by the International Council of Ophthalmology, 1954)

Decimal V Notation	6 metre Equivalent	20 feet Equivalent	Visual Angle (minutes)
1.0	6/6	20/20	1.0
0.9	–	–	1.1
0.8	5/6	20/25	1.3
0.7	6/9	20/30	1.4
0.6	5/9	15/25	1.6
0.5	6/12	20/40	2.0
0.4	5/12	20/50	2.5
0.3	6/18	20/70	3.3
0.2	–	–	5.0
0.1	6/60	20/200	10.0

In some countries, patients with less than 6/60 vision are classified as legally blind. Patients who can see 6/12 have sufficient vision to work in most industries and are said to have "industrial vision" which is also the visual requirement for driving.

Pinhole

In testing distant visual acuity, looking through a pinhole is useful for patients with blurred vision. Vision can be improved if the defective vision is due to refractive error. It cannot be improved if it is due to organic eye disease.

Near visual acuity

The common visual acuity tests are the Jaegar test and the 'N' chart, usually read at a distance of 30 cm. The Jaegar test is recorded as J1, J2, J4, J6, etc, and the 'N' chart as N5, N6, N8, N10, etc. Standard small newsprint is approximately J4 or N6. Each eye is tested in turn with the other covered. Middle-aged patients (presbyopic age) must be tested with their reading glasses.

Difficulties in examination

It is often difficult to test visual acuity in young children as well as patients who are illiterate, uncooperative or malingering. Frequently only an estimate can be made. The E-chart, picture cards or small coloured objects may be used. It can be extremely difficult to determine whether a patient is malingering without the use of special tests.

VISUAL FIELDS

Confrontation

The visual fields can be recorded approximately by using the confrontation test. The patient covers the eye which is not being tested with his palm and fixes the other at the examiner's nose, ear or eye. A target is then brought into his field of vision from the side and the point at which the patient sees the object is noted. The eye is tested in the different meridians, usually 8.

Alternatively, the examiner's fingers are held at a distance of one metre and the patient is asked to count them in the different quadrants, that is, the superior temporal, the inferior temporal, the superior nasal and the inferior nasal quadrants.

EXTERNAL EYE EXAMINATION

This is done with good illumination from either a window or a bright torch. A magnifying glass facilitates examination and should be used whenever available.

The position and appearance of the eyelids should be noted, especially their position in relation to the limbus, and whether there is eyelash crusting, watering, oedema, discharge or inflammation.

The conjunctiva and sclera should be almost white with only a few small vessels. The transparent disc-like cornea is best seen with either a good oblique light from a torch or window. Staining with fluorescein dye will help to show ulcers or abrasions of the cornea. The fluorescein is highlighted by blue light. The colour and pattern of the iris should be observed. A dense cataract can be seen through the pupil as a white reflex.

Eversion of upper eyelid

It is sometimes necessary to evert the upper lid to examine the tarsal conjunctiva if the patient is suspected of having a foreign body under the lid. This is also done for diagnosis of the conjunctival follicles of the upper lid as in trachoma. The lid is everted by asking the patient to look downwards and by applying slight pressure on the lid with a finger or rod. The lid margin is then gently pulled upwards to evert it.

PUPIL RESPONSES

The response of light directed at one pupil in a darkened room is known as the direct pupillary response. The reaction to light by the fellow pupil is called the consensual pupillary response.

Where a darkened room is not available, the pupillary response can be tested by having the patient cover both his eyes with his palms. The contraction of the pupil is observed when the palm is removed from one eye. This indicates the response of the pupil to direct light.

If there is no pupillary reaction to light, the reaction to accommodation is tested by asking the patient to fix on an object at a distance and then to focus on another object at about 10 cm from him.

EXTRAOCULAR MUSCLES

The extraocular muscles are examined by observing the position of the eyeballs with the patient looking straight ahead. Any gross malposition of the eyes can be easily seen. One eye may be observed to be turned inwards (convergent squint) or outwards (divergent squint). Occasionally, one of the eyes may be seen to be higher than the other (vertical squint).

Corneal light reflex

The corneal light reflex is a useful method of determining whether one of the eyes is turned inwards or outwards, or vertically displaced. Normally, when the patient is asked to look at a torch, a light reflex is seen at the centre of the pupil. If one of the eyes is misaligned, the reflex will not be at the centre of the pupil. In a convergent squint, the light reflex will be at the outer side of the cornea, and in a divergent squint, at the inner side of the cornea. A general guide is that if the reflex is at the limbus, the degree of convergence or divergence is approximately 40°. If it is halfway between the centre of the cornea and the limbus, it is approximately 20°. The corneal light reflex is also a useful means to exclude pseudosquints where there is an appearance of a convergent squint because of medial epicanthi lid folds. In pseudosquints the corneal light reflex is central in both eyes.

Ocular movements

When the extraocular muscles are severely paralysed, the restriction in movement is tested by asking the patient to look in different directions (positions of gaze). If the extraocular muscles are less severely affected, special techniques have to be used.

Movement	Right Eye	Left Eye
Right	Right lateral rectus	Left medial rectus
Up and right	Right superior rectus	Left inferior oblique
Down and right	Right inferior rectus	Left superior oblique
Left	Right medial rectus	Left lateral rectus
Up and left	Right inferior oblique	Left superior rectus
Down and left	Right superior oblique	Left inferior rectus

The six cardinal positions of gaze and their corresponding primary extraocular muscle actions.

OPHTHALMOSCOPY

The ophthalmoscope is used to observe abnormality in the ocular media, the optic disc, the retinal vessels, the fundal background and the macula.

Red reflex

With the lens power of the ophthalmoscope turned to 0 and the ophthalmoscope held a metre from the patient's eye a red reflex is seen through the pupil. Alternatively the lens power can be turned to about +5 dioptres and the eye examined approximately 10 cm away. This is caused by the reflection of the light of the ophthalmoscope from the choroidal vessels. It appears as a bright red round area which is evenly lighted. Any opacity in the cornea, lens (cataract) or vitreous will be seen as a dark area. In retinal detachment, the reflex appears grey instead of red.

Fundus

Examination of the fundus is usually done with the direct ophthalmoscope. The refractive error in both the patient and examiner has to be compensated for by adjusting the lens power of the ophthalmoscope. Alternatively, the examiner and patient may use their glasses or contact lenses in which case no adjustment will be required. The patient is then instructed to look at a distant object. When the right fundus is examined, the ophthalmoscope is held in the right hand. The examiner uses his right eye to examine the patient's right eye approaching from the right side. The patient's left fundus is examined with the examiner's left eye and the patient is approached from the left. It is important to get near enough so that the examiner's forehead touches his own thumb which is used to lift the upper lid of the eye being examined.

It is best to approach the eye from the temporal side so that a good view of the disc can be seen before the pupil contracts when light is shone on the macula. The nasal retinal vessels and the temporal retinal vessels are examined before the macula. Because of the extreme sensitivity of the macula to light which results in rapid constriction of the pupil, examination of the macula is difficult and usually requires a mydriatic eyedrop to dilate the pupil.

Difficulties in examination of the fundus

Examination of the fundus can be difficult because of:

- Uncooperative patient
- High myopia
- Opacity in the cornea, lens or vitreous
- Poor ophthalmoscope or old batteries
- Bright room
- Small pupils

In high myopia, examination is simplified by looking through the patient's glasses or his contact lenses. As the lenses of an ophthalmoscope can sometimes be fogged with dust or mould, especially in the tropics, they may have to be cleaned to enable adequate examination of the fundus.

The small pupil

In order to see the fundus clearly, the pupils should be dilated. Examination in a darkened room may be adequate for patients who have naturally large pupils. For patients with small pupils, examination can be difficult and a short-acting mydriatic such as Tropicamide, which acts in less than 30 minutes and has an effect of about four hours, should be used. Long-acting mydriatics are no longer used because of their length of action: Homatropine (one day) and Atropine (one week).

SPECIAL TECHNIQUES

Modern technology has enabled ophthalmologists to examine ocular conditions with greater precision. The techniques and equipment commonly used by ophthalmologists are described here to help other practitioners understand ophthalmic reports.

- **Tests for extraocular muscles**

The cover-uncover test is done by covering one of the patient's eyes while the other eye looks at an object. When the cover is removed, the uncovered eye may move to look at the object. By observing the movement of the eye, the presence of a squint may be confirmed.

A number of tests can be carried out to analyse diplopia with the use of red-green goggles to dissociate the eyes. The synoptophore is a machine with specially designed pictures to measure accurately the angle of a squint and to test the ability of the patient to see with both eyes together (binocular single vision).

- **Binocular slit-lamp microscopy**

The binocular slit-lamp microscope enables accurate observation of the eye up to a magnification of forty times. It consists of two parts, an oblique light which can be adjusted to a slit and a binocular microscope. Other uses of the slit-lamp include examination of the retina with magnification from a Hruby or contact lens and checking the filtrating angle of glaucoma patients (gonioscopy).

- **Tonometry**

A tonometer is used to measure intraocular pressure. The most widely used tonometer is the Goldmann Applanation Tonometer. The Schiotz Indentation Tonometer is less accurate but it is portable. The new non-contact tonometers do not require local anaesthesia.

- **Perimetry and scotometry**

Perimetry gives a more exact record of the visual fields than the confrontation test. The ability of the patient to see a small 5 mm target on an arc moving into his view from the periphery at different meridians is recorded on to a chart.

Scotometry is used to assess the central 30° part of the field of vision. It involves using a small 1-5 mm target on a screen (Bjerrum or Tangent screen) placed 1 or 2 metres away and noting when the test target appears. The normal blind spot is found 15° lateral to the fixation point.

- **Tests for colour vision**

The Ishihara charts are the most commonly used tests for colour vision. They are very sensitive. Patients who are able to see colours for general purposes may in fact be found to have a colour defect with it. Patients who fail the Ishihara chart but who respond accurately to the Lantern and other similar tests should not be prevented from pursuing their occupation of choice. This includes air pilots who generally need to have perfect or near perfect vision.

- **Indirect ophthalmoscopy**

The indirect ophthalmoscope is now commonly used by ophthalmologists. Its advantages are a binocular view, a wide field and easy examination of the retinal periphery. It is particularly valuable in assessing patients with opacity in the ocular media, high myopia and retinal detachment.

Fundal photography and fundal fluorescein angiography

Fundal photography and fundal fluorescein angiography are methods which supplement the examination of the fundus. In fundal fluorescein angiography, fluorescein dye is injected intravenously and serial fundal photographs are taken to show up the retinal and choroidal circulation.

Refraction

It can be objective with retinoscopy. Subjective tests are done with a trial frame and a set of lenses. Alternatively the lenses may be mounted on a series of rotating discs (phoropter). More recently, computerised scanning machines print out the refraction with remarkable accuracy.

Ultrasonography

Ultrasonography is now commonly used to evaluate the state of the posterior segment of the eyeball when the ocular media is opaque from corneal opacities, dense cataract or vitreous haemorrhage. It is particularly useful in severe ocular injuries and vitreous haemorrhage prior to posterior vitrectomy. Ultrasonography is also used for measuring the thickness of the cornea (pachymeter) and the axial length of the eye. In addition, it can provide essential data for calculating the required lens power prior to intraocular lens implanation in cataract extraction.

CT scan

This investigation is used for many ophthalmic conditions, but especially for orbital tumours and localisation of intraocular foreign bodies. It is also widely used for investigations of neuro-ophthalmic disorders.

Electrophysiology

Clinical electrophysiology which includes electroretinography (ERG), electrooculography (EOG) and visual evoked response study (VER) is now available in small practical units for ophthalmic clinics. ERG is useful in the diagnosis of retinal dystrophy, such as retinitis pigmentosa. It is also valuable in vitreous haemorrhage when the surgeon is unsure of visual function. EOG measures retinal pigment epithelial function, and VER is diminished in optic nerve disease.

Visual Acuity

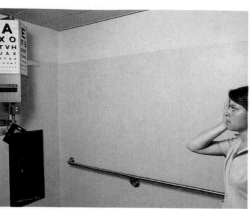

Fig. 1.1
Distant visual acuity examined at 6 m.

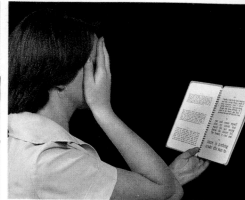

Fig. 1.2
Near visual acuity examined at about 30 cm.

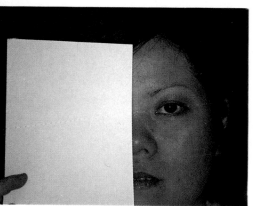

Fig. 1.3
Cardboard prevents patient from looking through slits between fingers.

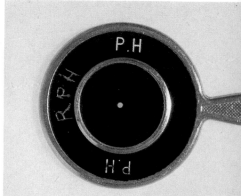

Fig. 1.4
Pinhole.

Examination of Anterior Segment

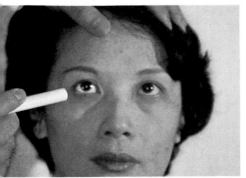

Fig. 1.5
Good focal illumination with oblique pocket torchlight.

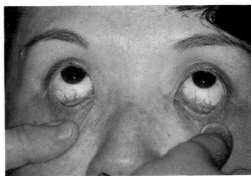

Fig. 1.6
Lower lids pulled down with patient looking up for examination of lower conjunctival fornix.

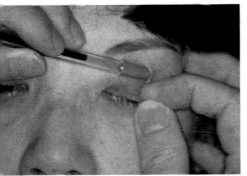

Fig. 1.7
Eversion of upper lid.

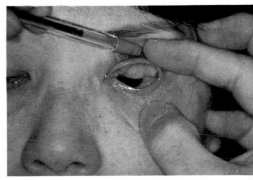

Fig. 1.8
Everted upper tarsal conjunctiva.

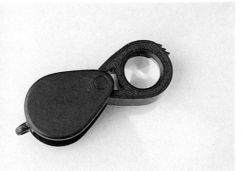

Fig. 1.9
Ordinary magnifier helps identify abnormalities.

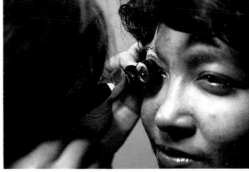

Fig. 1.10
Examination with magnifier and torch.

Extraocular Muscles

Corneal reflexes at centre of pupils signify normal ocular (alignments) muscle balance.

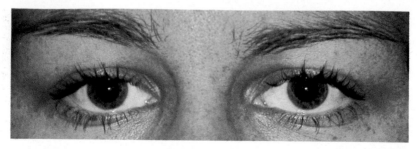

Fig. 1.11
Looking straight ahead.

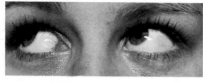

Fig. 1.12
Up and right. Right superior rectus and left inferior oblique

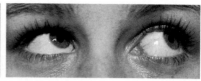

Fig. 1.13
Up and left. Right inferior oblique and left superior rectus.

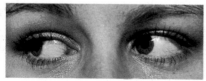

Fig. 1.14
Right. Right lateral rectus and left medial rectus.

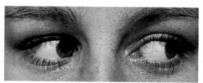

Fig. 1.15
Left. Right medial rectus and left lateral rectus.

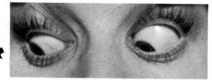

Fig. 1.16
Down and right. Right inferior rectus and left superior oblique.

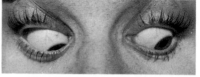

Fig. 1.17
Down and left. Right superior oblique and left inferior rectus.

Six cardinal positions of gaze and their corresponding primary extraocular muscle actions.

Red Reflex

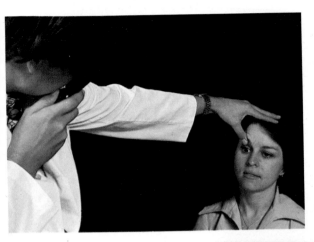

Fig. 1.18
Examination of red reflex at 1 m
using (direct) ophthalmoscope.

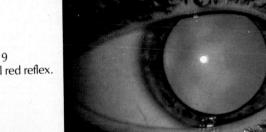

Fig. 1.19
Normal red reflex.

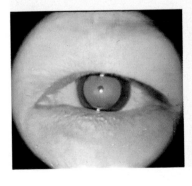

Fig. 1.20
Red reflex with central opacity.

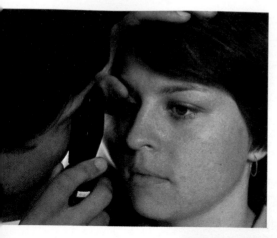

Fig. 1.21
Right fundus examined with right eye of examiner from right side of patient.

Fig. 1.22
Normal fundus in Caucasians.

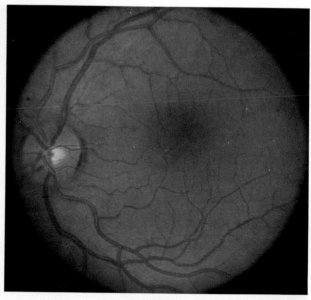

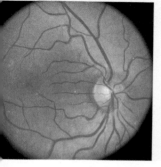

Fig. 1.23
Normal fundus in pigmented races.

DESCRIPTION OF THE FUNDUS

Optic disc

Colour — Pink, temporal side usually paler.

Margin — Sharp and flat. Nasal margin may be relatively blurred and raised (in hypermetropia). Many normal variations including pigmentation and myopic crescent.

Cup — Varies in size and depth. Situated at centre of disc and slopes temporally.

Cup/disc ratio — is ratio of diameter of cup and that of optic disc.

Retinal vessels

Colour — Arteries lighter than veins.

Diameter — Arteries narrower than veins. Ratio approximately 2:3.

Crossing — Arteries cross anterior to veins at arterio-venous crossings.

Fundus background

Colour — Red fundal background because of the choroidal vessels and retinal pigment layer. Darker in pigmented races. In lightly pigmented persons, large choroidal vessels seen against the white sclera. Tesselated (tigroid appearance) in myopia.

Macular area

Colour — Normally darker than rest of fundus. At centre, normal foveal light reflex.

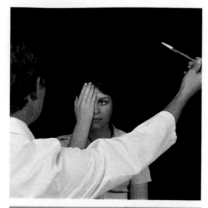

Fig. 1.24
Visual fields by confrontation. Patient looks at examiner's right ear while test object is moved in from periphery.

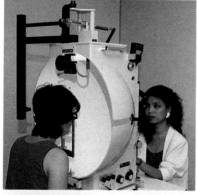

Fig. 1.25
Perimetry permits accurate record of peripheral visual fields.

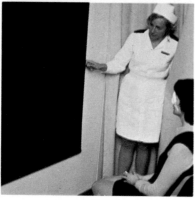

Fig. 1.26
Central fields (30° from fixation spot) tested on tangent screen using scotometer.

Visual Field Charts

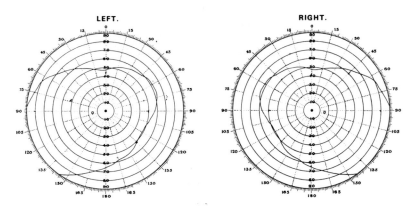

Fig. 1.27
Perimetry chart.

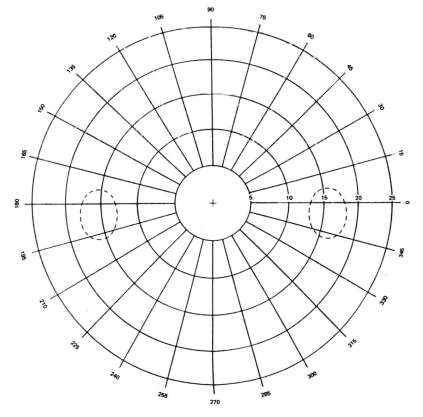

Fig. 1.28
Central field chart.

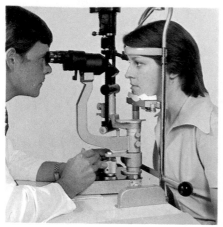

Fig. 1.29
Slit-lamp microscopy permits not only magnified examination of anterior segment but also flitration angles, intraocular pressure with applanation tonometer, vitreous and retina with special contact lens.

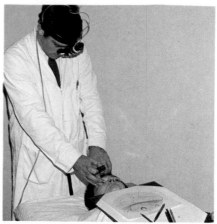

Fig. 1.30
Indirect ophthalmoscopy permits good binocular examination of retinal periphery, especially useful in retinal detachment or cloudy media.

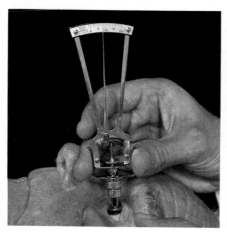

Fig. 1.31
Schiotz tonometry, one of the methods of measuring intraocular pressure.

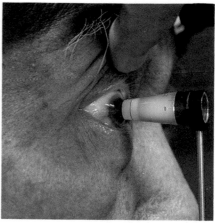

Fig. 1.32
Applanation tonometry using fluorescein and blue cobalt light is most accurate method of measuring intraocular pressure.

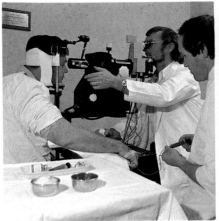

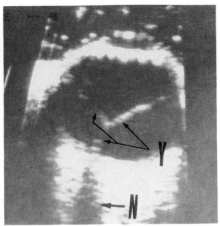

Fig. 1.33
Fundal photography with intravenous fluorescein dye injection (fundal fluorescein angiography).

Fig. 1.34
Ultrasonography now extensively used in ophthalmology especially when ocular medium is opaque (note total retinal detachment).

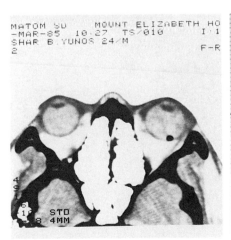

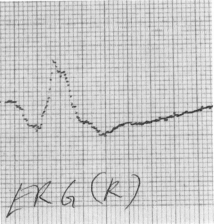

Fig. 1.35
CT scan useful in numerous conditions. Helps to confirm diagnosis of intraocular foreign body (note intraocular foreign body near optic disc).

Fig. 1.36
Electrophysiological studies now used clinically in many retinal conditions.

2

LID, LACRIMAL APPARATUS AND ORBIT

INTRODUCTION

Most lid conditions are related to inflammation, malposition or tumours. A common lacrimal disease is blockage of the lacrimal drainage system which results in tearing.

The most common condition of the orbit is exophthalmos, indicating the possibility of thyroid disease or a space-occupying lesion. It may require the care of several specialists.

EYELID INFLAMMATION

Blepharitis (inflammation of the lid margin)

Squamous blepharitis is the more common of the two main types of blepharitis. It is frequently associated with dandruff or seborrheic dermatitis and presents with small white scales at the roots of the eyelashes. The patient often has chronically irritable eyes.

Ulcerative blepharitis is due to staphylococcal infection of the follicles at the lid margin. It is accompanied by the falling of the lashes and, later, by deformity of the lashes, some of which may turn inwards (trichiasis).

Treatment is frequently difficult and tedious as the condition is chronic. The crusts may be removed by cleaning the lid margins with boiled cotton wool, followed by the application of an antibiotic ointment at night. It is best to avoid local steroids although they may relieve the symptoms. In squamous blepharitis, scalp lotion to control the dandruff may help.

Stye (hordeolum)

This is a small abscess of the eyelash follicle seen clinically as a small inflamed nodule. The symptoms are acute irritation and local pain. Treatment is with local heat applied with a folded face towel. If the abscess points, the affected eyelash may be pulled out and local antibiotics applied.

Chalazion (Meibomian cyst)

Blockage of the duct of a tarsal gland may cause a cyst (Meibomian cyst) due to the retained secretion. This is sometimes inflamed and is often successfully treated with local heat and local antibiotics. Systemic antibiotics are rarely necessary. Surgery may be necessary if the cyst is large, becomes inflamed or ruptures, resulting in a granulomatous lesion on the conjunctiva or skin.

Allergic or contact dermatitis

The skin around the eyelids becomes oedematous, inflamed and scaly. There is intense itching. This is due to allergy to cosmetics or a variety of ophthalmic medication, especially sulphonamides.

Treatment consists of identifying and stopping the offending cosmetics or medication. The application of local steroid cream to the skin of the eyelids helps

Herpes zoster ophthalmicus

Herpes zoster ophthalmicus affects the skin supplied by the ophthalmic division of the fifth cranial nerve. It presents with pain and skin vesicles which may become secondarily infected. If the nasociliary nerve is affected, the skin lesions appear on one side of the nose. In this case the eye is at risk from complications which include corneal inflammation, iridocyclitis and occasionally, secondary glaucoma.

Treatment consists of providing general hygiene and the application of local antibiotics to prevent secondary infection of the skin lesion. Application of local steroids to the eye is needed if keratitis or iridocyclitis develops. Ocular complications may require regular ophthalmic care. Systemic antiviral drugs may be indicated in severe cases during the acute stage. Prolonged pain over the scalp and eye (post- herpetic neuralgia) may be troublesome.

EYELID MALPOSITION

Ptosis (drooping upper lid)

Ptosis can be unilateral or bilateral, complete or partial, and congenital or acquired. In bilateral ptosis, the patient's head is characteristically tilted backwards in order to see through the narrowed palpebral fissure.

The causes of acquired ptosis include muscle abnormality in myasthenia gravis, third nerve lesion, trauma to the lid, Horner's syndrome and inflammation. Occasionally, senile ptosis may occur.

Treatment for congenital ptosis consists of an operation to shorten the levator palpebrae superioris, usually with good cosmetic results. Treatment for other types of ptosis depends on the cause.

Lid retraction

Instead of covering the upper edge of the cornea, the upper lid is retracted several millimetres. The usual cause is overactivity of the levator muscle from hyperthyroidism. In severe cases, a recession of the levator muscle may be done.

Control of hyperthyroidism may be helpful. In severe cases, a plastic bridging of the lids (tarsorrhaphy) or alternatively, a recession of the levator muscle may be done.

Entropion (inversion of lid margin)

This condition is associated with inturned eyelashes (trichiasis) which may lead to complications including chronic conjunctivitis, corneal abrasion and even ulceration.

The cause may be scar tissue on the conjunctival surface, a common complication of the end stage of trachoma, or spasm of the orbicularis oculi (spastic entropion). It may also be due to weakness of the eyelid tissues as in senile entropion.

Lubricants may help but surgical eversion of the lid is usually required.

Trichiasis (inturned eyelashes)

Trichiasis can cause a unilateral red eye from chronic irritation of the cornea or conjunctiva. It is frequently associated with entropion. For a permanent cure, the hair follicles of the inturned lashes have to be destroyed by diathermy or cryotherapy. Alternatively, the eyelid may be everted surgically.

Ectropion (eversion of lid margin)

The patient usually complains of tearing (epiphora) due to failure of the tears to gain access to the lacrimal drainage apparatus. This is sometimes accompanied by exposure conjunctivitis or keratitis.

The cause of ectropion is weakness of the orbicularis oculi muscles associated with seventh nerve lesion or senile weakness from loss of muscle tone. Occasionally, it is caused by scar tissue on the skin of the eyelid (cicatricial ectropion).

When the watering is disturbing or when it is complicated by exposure conjunctivitis or keratitis, a plastic operation may be necessary to restore the lid to its normal position.

EYELID DEPOSITS & TUMOUR

Xanthelasma

Xanthelasma is a fatty deposit in the skin, usually bilateral and occurring at the medial part of the upper lid. Less commonly, it develops on the lower lid. It is a local condition which has no symptoms. Surgical removal is for cosmetic reason.

Basal-cell carcinoma (rodent ulcer)

Basal cell carcinoma usually appears on the lower lid margin as a raised nodule with a characteristic pearly rolled edge. This is common in Caucasians living in hot climates. If left untreated, the lesion may ulcerate and infiltrate into the adjacent tissues. It may, although rarely, lead to loss of the eye or the invasion of the bone and may even reach the surface of the brain. The lesion is locally invasive and does not metastasize.

The choice of treatment is between surgery and radiotherapy. Careful follow-up is essential in order to prevent recurrence.

Blockage of the lacrimal drainage system may occur either in the punctum, the canaliculus or the naso-lacrimal duct, resulting in tearing. Very often, the blockage occurs in the nasolacrimal duct and this secretion may cause the lacrimal sac to become chronically infected (chronic dacryocystitis). The patient complains of persistent watering in the eye with reflux of muco-purulent material when pressure is applied on the lacrimal sac.

If the condition persists, an operation (dacryocystorhinostomy) to create a new drainage channel may have to be performed. In acute dacryocystitis, systemic antibiotics and surgical drainage of the pus are required.

ORBIT

Orbital cellulitis

This condition is unilateral. It presents with intense lid oedema, chemosis and restriction of the eye movements. It often occurs as a result of the spread of infection to the orbit from one of the surrounding paranasal sinuses. Sometimes there is disc oedema.

The infection may spread backwards and cause cavernous sinus thrombosis, a condition which can be fatal. The patient usually has systemic manifestations of fever and malaise.

Treatment is urgent. Intensive medication with systemic antibiotics usually clears the infection. X-ray of the sinuses should be taken and an ear, nose and throat specialist consulted.

Exophthalmos (proptosis or forward protrusion of the eyeball)

This is recognised clinically by the position of the lower lid margin which normally just covers the limbus but which is separated away in exophthalmos. The protrusion is sometimes more obvious when the patient is examined from above and the positions of both eyes are compared.

Thyroid disease is the commonest cause. Other causes include space-occupying lesion behind the eyeball which may arise from orbital structures or which may have spread from the middle cranial fossa or the posterior nasal space. It may also be caused by metastatic tumours.

It is important to distinguish exophthalmos from pseudo-exophthalmos which occurs in lid retraction (hyperthyroidism) and in myopia when the eyes may appear to protrude forward.

Owing to the variety of causes, investigations often involve the neurologists, the endocrinologist, the radiologist and the ear, nose and throat surgeon.

Treatment depends on the cause. A local intraocular space-occupying lesion may require surgical removal. If the cornea is at risk, it needs protection, usually a tarsorrhaphy.

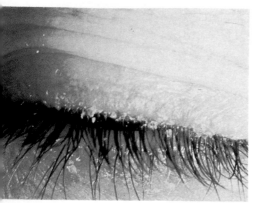

Fig. 2.1
Squamous blepharitis (crusting at base of lashes).

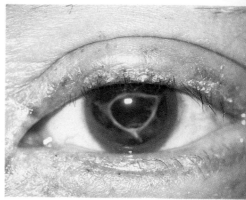

Fig. 2.2
Ulcerative blepharitis.

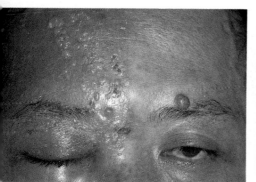

Fig. 2.3
Herpes zoster ophthalmicus with vesicles affecting upper eyelid and forehead.

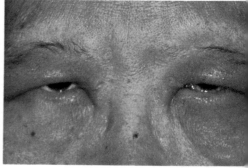

Fig. 2.4
Allergic dermatitis resulting from sulphacetamide eyedrops.

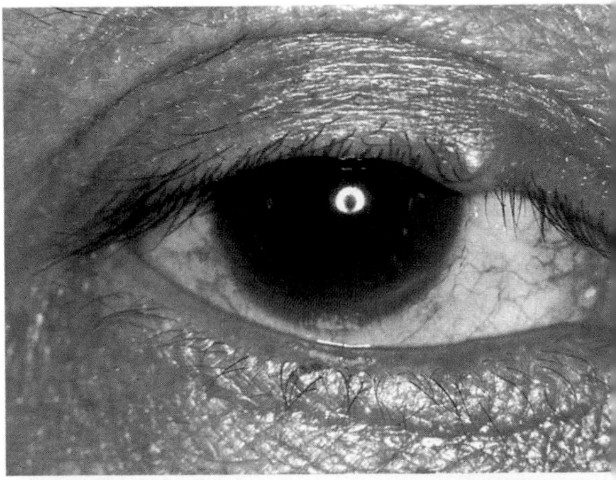

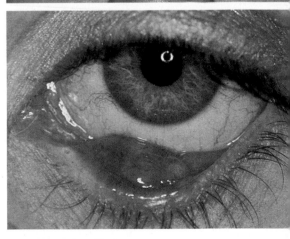

Fig. 2.5
Stye (abscess of eyelash follicle).

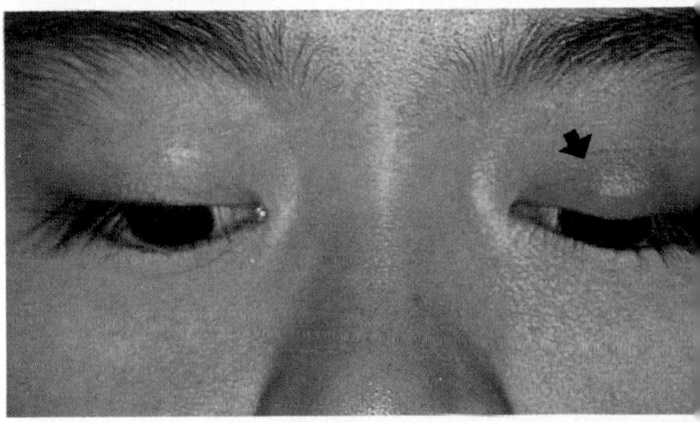

Fig. 2.6
Inflamed chalazion of left upper lid.

Fig. 2.7
Infected chalazion ruptured through conjunctiva and appearing as granulomatous lesion.

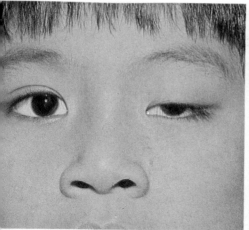

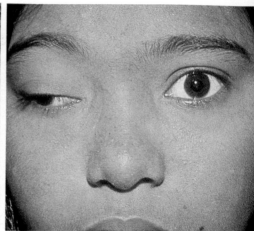

Fig. 2.8
Left congenital ptosis (drooping of eyelid).

Fig. 2.9
Right ptosis from third nerve paralysis. Pupil dilated and eye displaced (turned down and out).

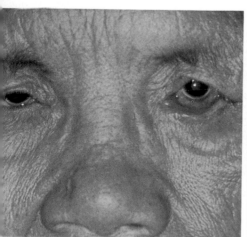

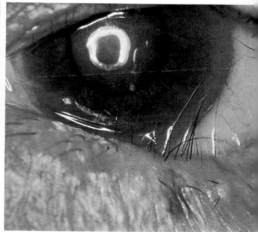

Fig. 2.10
Ectropion of left lower lid (eversion of eyelid) with exposure keratitis.

Fig. 2.11
Entropion (inturned eyelid) with trichiasis (inturned lashes).

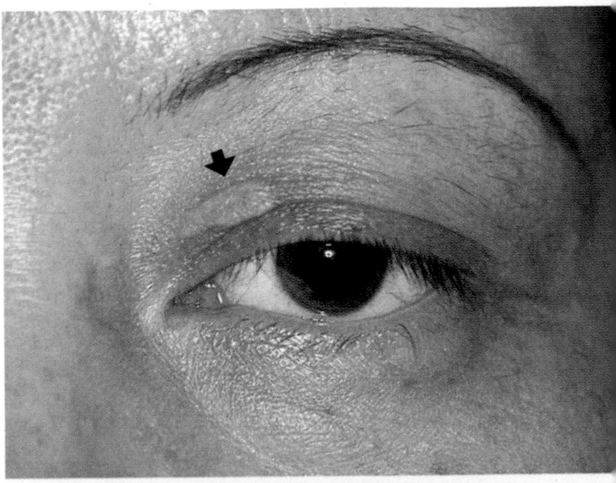

Deposits and Tumour of Eyelid

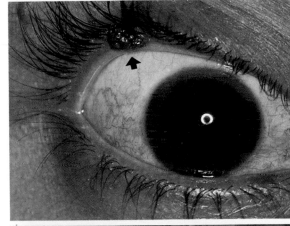

Fig. 2.12
Xanthelasma (fatty deposits on eyelid).

Fig. 2.13
Benign melanoma at upper eyelid margin.

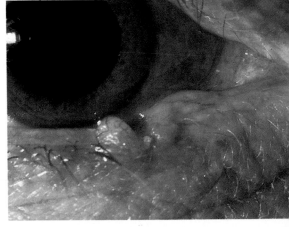

Fig. 2.14
Basal-cell carcinoma at lid margin with central ulcer and raised edges.

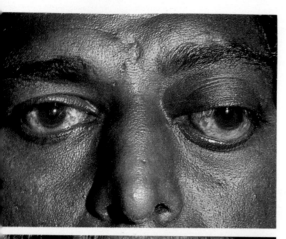

Fig. 2.15
Left exophthalmos caused by retrobulbar tumour (note left lower lid 4 mm away from limbus).

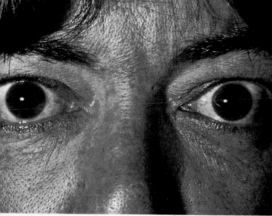

Fig. 2.16
Exophthalmos with lid retraction in thyroid exophthalmos.

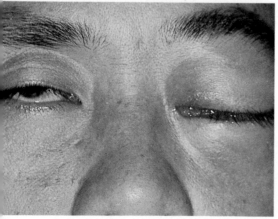

Fig. 2.17
Left orbital cellulitis with lid oedema and chemosis (oedema of conjunctiva).

3

CONJUNCTIVA SCLERA AND CORNEA

INTRODUCTION

Bilateral red eyes from infection or allergy are common and relatively harmless. However, a unilateral red eye requires careful ocular examination as the common causes are acute glaucoma, acute iritis, keratitis, or a foreign body. These conditions can lead to blindness if untreated.

Corneal diseases may lead to visual loss because of scarring. Of particular importance are trachoma and herpes simplex infection. Corneal graft surgery may restore vision to patients with central corneal opacities.

BILATERAL RED EYES

Bacterial conjunctivitis

Acute bacterial conjunctivitis is a common cause of bilateral red eyes. It presents with a history of discharge and sticky eyelids, especially in the morning. The sensation of grittiness or of having a foreign body in the eyes is due to the rubbing of the inflamed palpebral conjunctiva against the cornea. The diagnosis is usually straightforward especially when it occurs during an epidemic. Intensive application of local antibiotic eyedrops every three hours should cure the condition. It is, however, important to continue with the eyedrops for two days after the infection has cleared clinically. At night, an antibiotic ointment may be used for prolonged effect and to prevent stickiness of the lids in the morning.

Padding of the eyes should be avoided as it tends to aggravate the infection. If the condition does not improve in forty-eight hours, treatment should be reviewed. Bacteriological swabs and cultures may then be helpful.

Viral conjunctivitis

Viral conjunctivitis presents with bilateral watering red eyes. The discharge is less than that in bacterial conjunctivitis. Sometimes, the eyes are irritable and photophobic, owing to an associated keratitis which may lead to blurred vision. The virus may also cause preauricular and submandibular lymphadenopathy. A fever or upper respiratory infection may be associated. There is no specific treatment. When there is corneal involvement, steroids can be used under slit-lamp control. To prevent bacterial infection, antibiotics may help.

Preventive measures, especially washing the hands after examining each patient, must be taken during epidemics. Patients should wash their hands, and handkerchiefs and hand towels should not be shared. The family should be kept apart during the acute stage.

Allergic conjunctivitis

Allergic conjunctivitis presents with intense itchiness, in addition to watering red eyes. Sometimes it is associated with vasomotor-rhinitis or a history of allergies such as rashes, reaction to drugs or cosmetics and hay fever.

Treatment with a decongestive or antihistamine eyedrop combined with oral antihistamine is usually effective. Steroids should not be used except in the occasional severe cases.

Spring catarrh (vernal conjunctivitis)

A specific allergic conjunctivitis which is less common is spring catarrh. It is usually seasonal, mostly affecting boys. Large flat papillary conjunctival thickenings form on the upper tarsal conjunctiva. Corti-costeroid eyedrops give relief. Corneal complications occasionally develop.

Chronic non-specific conjunctivitis

Chronic non-specific conjunctivitis is a condition presenting with a multitude of symptoms which include a sensation of dryness, discomfort, irritation, burning, redness, and sometimes, watering and pain as well. The eyes are constantly irritable particularly when exposed to irritants which include bright sunlight, dust, smoke, airconditioning and wind.

Examination usually shows no abnormality. Investigations should be carried out to exclude specific causes such as inturned lashes (trichiasis), defective tear flow (dry-eye), chronic allergy or eyelid infection (blepharitis).

Treatment depends on identification of contributory factors and use of artificial tears, antihistamine drops and sometimes weak vasoconstrictors. Antibiotics and steroids should not be used. The condition tends to persist despite treatment and patient requires frequent reassurance.

UNILATERAL RED EYE

A unilateral red eye is a potentially dangerous condition. It may be due to serious ocular conditions such as acute closed-angle glaucoma, iritis, keratitis, corneal ulcer or a foreign body. Less commonly it is due to scleritis. Of particular importance is acute closed-angle glaucoma which presents with a unilateral red eye associated with headache, pain in the eye or blurred vision. Prompt consultation with an ophthalmologist is required.

Unilateral conjunctivitis is usually due to an underlying cause such as a blocked nasolacrimal duct or trichiasis (inturned eyelashes). It is important to carry out a thorough investigation of a unilateral red eye to establish the cause.

Subconjunctival haemorrhage

This condition also presents as a unilateral red eye. Rubbing of the eyes and severe coughing may cause capillary rupture resulting in haemorrhage into the subconjunctival space. It is sometimes spontaneous.

No treatment is normally required except to reassure the patient that the haemorrhage will take one to two weeks to absorb. Occasionally, the condition recurs. If it does, investigations to exclude blood dyscrasia may be carried out.

TRACHOMA

This is a major world-wide blinding condition caused by infection brought about by an organism known as "chlamydia trachomatis". It has a varying pattern in different countries. In developed societies it is benign and oculo-genital in origin. In less developed countries, it is endemic with up to 90% of some populations showing signs of trachoma. In some areas 10% of those infected become blind. It is not entirely clear why the organism behaves differently in different environments.

The clinical features vary considerably. At the initial stage, it may be asymptomatic, or may present with acute conjunctivitis. The signs of active infection are white, round follicles on the conjunctival surface of the upper lids associated with a velvety papillary hypertrophy. Follicles at the limbus leave small depressions known as Herbert's pits, which are permanent diagnostic signs of previous trachoma. A layer of new blood vessels and connective tissue (pannus) usually invades the upper cornea. Healing leads to scars. If compounded by cyclical reinfection and superimposed bacterial infection, entropion (inturned eyelid), trichiasis (inturned eyelashes) and blindness due to opaque cornea or even endophthalmitis may result.

In active trachoma, local broad spectrum antibiotics such as tetracycline may be repeated twice a day for six weeks. This may be combined with oral broad spectrum antibiotics or oral sulphonamides. If mass surveys reveal that over 20% of the population are actively infected, treatment is given to the whole population to eliminate the infectious pool of chlamydia.

Surgical correction of entropion and trichiasis relieves discomfort and decreases the risk of visual loss from corneal scarring and infection. If there is corneal scarring, it is sometimes possible to improve vision with corneal graft surgery.

In spite of advances in modern medicine, trachoma remains one of the most difficult eye diseases to eradicate in developing countries mainly because of poor and unhygienic living conditions which include lack of water supply, dust and flies. These encourage cyclical reinfection and superimposed bacterial infection.

RAISED CONJUNCTIVAL LESIONS

Pinguecula

This is a tiny, cream-coloured, slightly raised opaque lesion on the conjunctiva, usually on the nasal side of the cornea but sometimes on the temporal side. The pinguecula usually causes no symptoms. It is common in the tropics, and may be related to exposure to the sun. No treatment is required except for reassurance that it is not a growth. Surgical removal for cosmetic reason is seldom required.

Pterygium

Pterygium is a triangular fleshy wing of conjunctiva which encroaches on the cornea usually on the nasal side. Some pterygia are vascular, thick and fleshy while others are avascular and flat. It is usually bilateral and harmless but may cause mild astigmatism. In rare cases, visual disturbance may result from the spread of the pterygium across the pupillary area. This condition is common in the tropics and is associated with exposure to the sun.

Simple excision by a variety of methods may be considered if the pterygium encroaches on the cornea by 3 mm or more. Recurrence is high in some countries (50%). To prevent recurrence, betatherapy with strontium 90 or thiotepa eyedrops may be applied with great care. Betatherapy in doses of 2,000 rads or more may cause scleral necrosis.

Conjunctival melanoma (naevus)

Benign conjunctival melanoma is a common harmless condition. The lesion occasionally grows in size during puberty. It may be removed for cosmetic reasons. Malignant conjunctival melanoma is uncommon.

CORNEAL ULCER

Corneal ulcers are usually due to the herpes simplex virus infection, bacterial infection or trauma.

Herpes simplex dendritic ulcer

Herpes simplex dendritis ulcer is a serious infection of the cornea caused by the herpes simplex virus. The eye is usually irritable, red, watering and photophobic.

A typical branched dendritic ulcer usually develops. Sometimes, there are complications such as disciform keratitis, a deep stromal, disc-like inflammation of the cornea and iritis. The condition tends to recur especially during periods of stress or fever. A number of antiviral agents, such as Idoxuridine, are specific against the virus. In some cases, the infected loose epithelium may be removed with either a cotton bud after application of Amethocaine eyedrops, or by the use of some other mechanical or chemical method. Steroid eyedrops are absolutely contra-indicated, as they lead to serious corneal complications or even perforation of the eye. They should be avoided even when the condition is quiet as they can precipitate an attack of the infection.

Bacterial corneal ulcer

The signs and symptoms are those of a unilateral red eye which is painful, watering and photophobic. The vision is blurred. It is caused by bacterial infection from a variety of organisms. Pneumococcus and pseudomonas pyocyaneus are serious infections which lead to large destructive corneal ulcers.Bacteriological studies are essential for precise diagnosis and treatment. The ulcer should be scrapped for examination with gram stain.

Treatment is urgent. It includes intensive application of broad-spectrum antibiotics usually Gentamycin and Cephalosporin locally and subconjunctivally. Systemic antibiotics is sometimes also required. Dilatation of the pupil with Atropine eyedrops prevents synechiae (iris adhesions) and subsequent glaucoma. Bacteriological studies are essential in severe cases.

Small marginal corneal ulcers

These are frequently associated with ulcerative blepharitis and are believed to be allergic to staphylococcus infection. Treatment with antibiotic eyedrops is effective and may be combined with steroids.

Severe corneal ulcers can often be prevented by adequate initial treatment of minor injuries. Application of drops of broad-spectrum antibiotics are particularly important in rural areas where ophthalmic care is not immediately available. Severe and neglected corneal ulcers lead to blindness from corneal scarring, corneal perforation, secondary glaucoma and panophthalmitis.

Fungus corneal ulcer

Corneal ulcers caused by a wide variety of fungi have a more insidious and protracted cause. They are particularly likely to occur in susceptible eyes with depressed immunity after prolonged treatment with steroid or antibiotic drops and in eyes after injury with organic material. Scrapings may reveal the fungus. Treatment is with local and sometimes systemic antifungal agents. Eradication is often difficult and corneal grafting may be required. Prognosis is poor.

CORNEAL OPACITY

If the corneal scarring is in the periphery, the vision remains good, but when it is central it can interfere severely with vision. Common causes are healed herpes keratitis, or ulcer trachoma, trauma and keratomalacia from Vitamin A deficiency. In many cases a corneal graft can restore vision.

Arcus senilis

This is a white ring at the periphery of the cornea, caused by lipid deposits at the limbal region. The central cornea is never affected. It is sometimes found in young adults (arcus juvenilis). The condition is harmless.

Corneal dystrophies

Corneal dystrophies affect both eyes symmetrically. Keratoconus is a dystrophic condition in young adults where the cornea becomes conical in shape. The patient becomes highly short-sighted with severe irregular astigmatism. Vision is initially improved with glasses. Later, contact lenses may help to improve vision considerably. But if the condition is advanced, contact lenses will not help. Corneal graft surgery is very effective.

Hereditary corneal dystrophies of various types cause minute opacities in the central cornea. Some will lead to severe visual loss in early life and may require corneal grafting.

Fuch's endothelial dystrophy presents with corneal oedema and opacity. It can lead to severe visual loss. It usually occurs in the middle-aged or the elderly and is more common in Caucasians than in Asians. It is caused by dystrophic changes in the corneal endothelium. Sometimes, it follows cataract extraction. Corneal graft surgery may help.

Non-ulcerative (interstitial) keratitis

In the active stage, interstitial keratitis is bilateral and presents itself as a patch of vessels with corneal opacity. In the later stages, the eye is quiet with residual opacity of varying intensity in the deep corneal layer and ghost vessels which are best seen under the slit-lamp microscope. Congenital syphilis is the usual cause.

The acute stage responds rapidly to local steroids. Antibiotics may be used if desired but the effect is usually insignificant. Defective vision due to corneal opacity can be improved with corneal graft surgery.

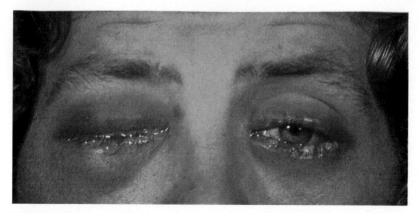

Fig. 3.1
Bilateral bacterial conjunctivitis with lid oedema and sticky mucopurulent discharge.

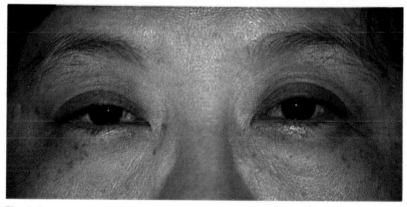

Fig. 3.2
Bilateral viral conjunctivitis with watering red eyes and little discharge.

Unilateral Red Eye

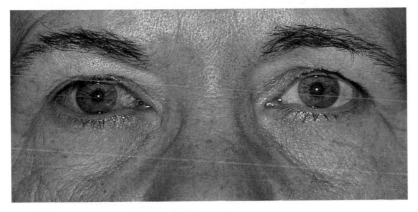

Fig. 3.3
Iritis presenting as unilateral red eye.

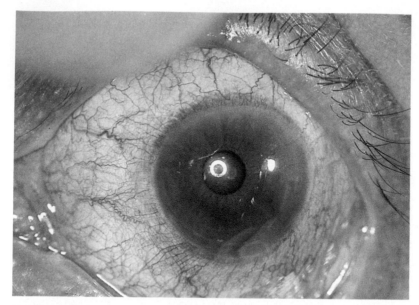

Fig. 3.4
Iritis presenting as red eye with small pupil.

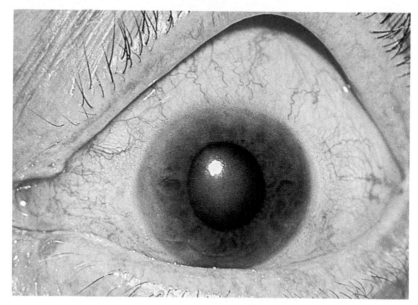

Fig. 3.5
Acute glaucoma presenting as red eye with fixed dilated pupil and corneal haze.

Dendritic Corneal Ulcers

Dendritic ulcer is major cause of severe visual loss from corneal disease in developed countries.

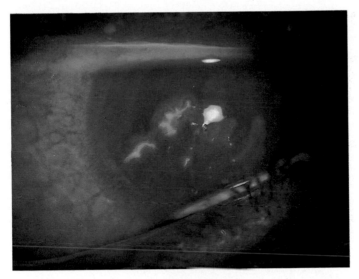

Fig. 3.6
Dendritic ulcer caused by herpes simplex virus. Ulcer best seen under magnification with fluorescein stain.

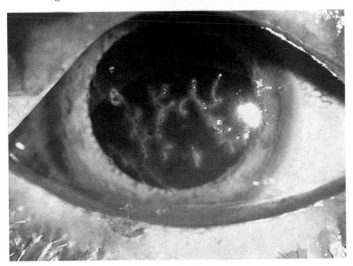

Fig. 3.7
Fluorescein stain of dendritic ulcer with numerous branches made worse by use of steroid eyedrops.

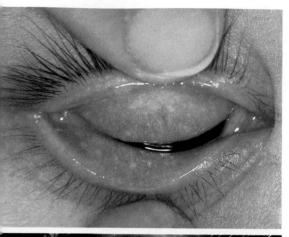

Fig. 3.8
Follicular conjunctivitis resulting from allergy. Follicles mainly on lower palpebral conjunctiva.

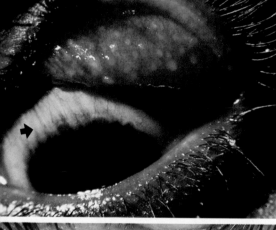

Fig. 3.9
Follicular conjunctivitis of trachoma. Follicles on upper palpebral conjunctiva. (Note diagnostic Herbert's pits at limbus).

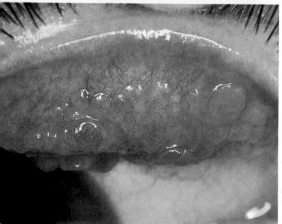

Fig. 3.10
Spring catarrh (vernal conjunctivitis) with large flattened papillary hypertrophy of upper palpebral conjunctiva, sometimes mistaken for trachomatous follicles.

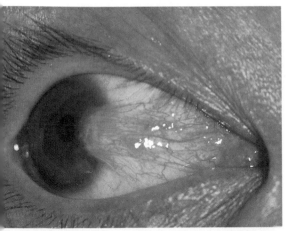

Fig. 3.11
Nasal pterygium encroaching on cornea.

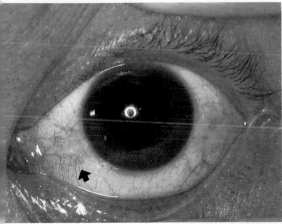

Fig. 3.12
Nasal pinguecula. (Note: cornea not affected).

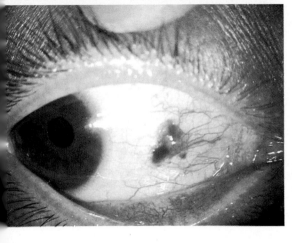

Fig. 3.13
Benign melanoma (naevus) of conjunctiva.

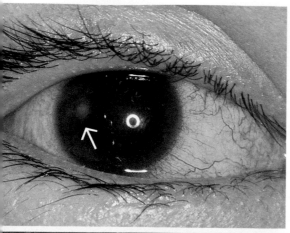

Fig. 3.14
Small corneal ulcer caused by staphylococcal infection from use of soft contact lens.

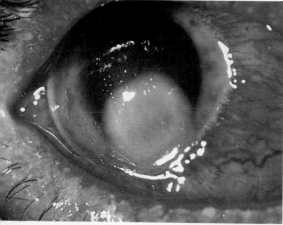

Fig. 3.15
Severe pseudomonas pyocyaneus corneal ulcer.

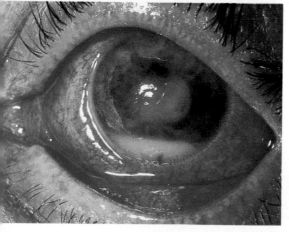

Fig. 3.16
Central pneumococcal corneal ulcer with hypopyon (pus in anterior chamber).

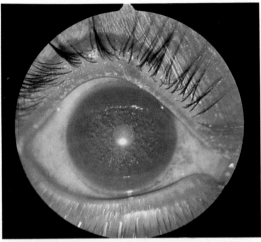

Fig. 3.17
Hereditary corneal dystrophy.

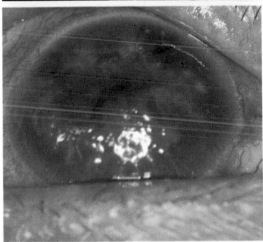

Fig. 3.18
Fuch's corneal dystrophy with diffuse corneal oedema.

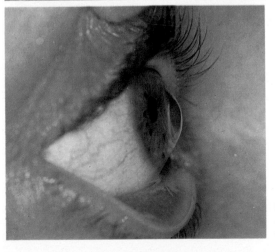

Fig. 3.19
Keratoconus with conical cornea and opacity at apex.

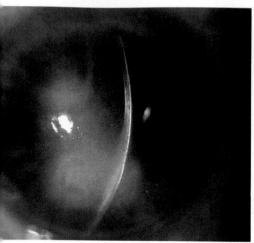

Fig. 3.20
Slit picture of interstitial keratitis showing stromal thickening, opacity with abnormal corneal vessels.

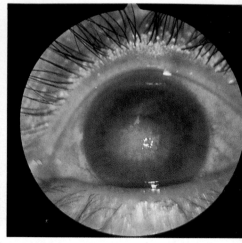

Fig. 3.21
Corneal opacity caused by herpes simplex infection (disciform keratitis).

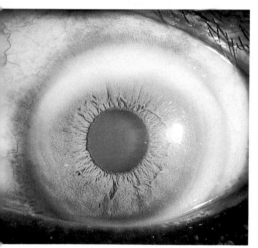

Fig. 3.22
Arcus senilis at corneal periphery. (Never affects vision).

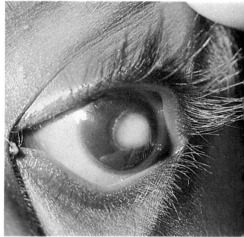

Fig. 3.23
Central corneal opacity following keratomalacia due to Vitamin A deficiency.

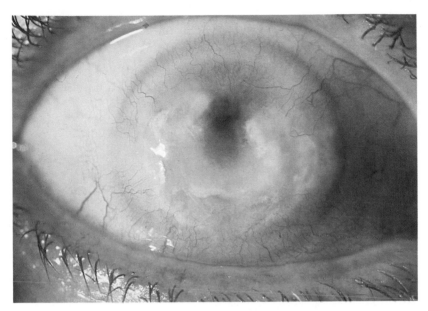

Fig. 3.24
Before surgery, dense corneal opacity causing blindness.

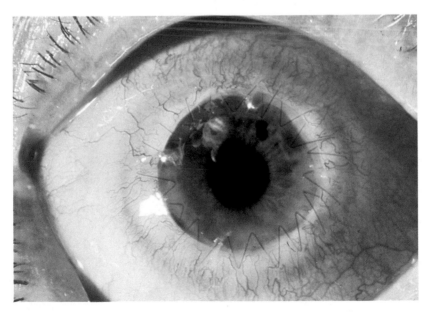

Fig. 3.25
After surgery, clear penetrating corneal graft with continuous 10/0 monofilament nylon suture.

4

LENS AND GLAUCOMA

INTRODUCTION

Cataract is a common cause of gradual painless visual loss in the elderly. The usual indication for surgery is when the patient's vision has deteriorated to such an extent that it interferes with his normal activities. Mature cataracts can lead to complications. Thick glasses are required after surgery but many patients are unable to tolerate them. This problem is overcome with intraocular implants. Contact lens is a less satisfactory alternative.

Glaucoma is a major cause of blindness. Open-angle (chronic) glaucoma is asymptomatic. Acute closed-angle glaucoma presents as a red eye associated with sudden visual loss, ocular pain and headache. It blinds an eye rapidly unless urgently and adequately treated.

CATARACT

A cataract is an opacity in the clear lens. Normally, the human lens converges light rays. An opacity in the lens will scatter or block the light rays. If the opacity is small and at the lens periphery, there will be little or no interference with vision. On the other hand, when the opacity is central and dense, the light rays can be severely interfered with. This will lead to blurred vision.

The most common cause of cataract is old age and this is known as senile cataract. Less common causes include damage to the lens by injury, drugs (steroids) and general diseases such as diabetes and hypo-parathyrodism.

Management

Timing for cataract surgery depends on the patient's visual requirements. Cataract extraction should be considered if a change of glasses cannot improve vision or when the patient's normal activities are seriously interfered with. However, cataract extraction is required if the cataract is mature as it can lead to complications. With the modern technique of early mobilisation, age and poor general health may not be a contraindication for surgery.

Surgical removal of cataract is by the intracapsular or extracapsular method. In intracapsular cataract extraction, the whole lens together with its capsule is removed. In extracapsular extraction, the nucleus and the cortex are removed through an opening in the anterior capsule (anterior capsulectomy) leaving the posterior capsule intact. It is the operation of choice in countries where modern technology, especially a good operating microscope, is available. An intraocular lens is now frequently inserted behind the iris (posterior chamber lens implant). Cataract removal by ultrasonic emulsification has few advantages.

With the aid of the operating microscope, the incision is made and sutured with precision. Patients are not required to be confined to bed for a long period. Most patients sit up or get out of bed and walk with help, as soon as they recover from the effects of anaesthesia or sedation. The period of hospitalisation usually does not exceed three days and many surgeons prefer cataract surgery performed as an outpatient procedure.

Cataract extraction is one of the most satisfying operations for both the surgeon and the patient. Most patients regain their eyesight or have a considerable improvement in vision following a successful extraction. Failure to restore normal vision is usually due to abnormality of the retina or the optic nerve.

Post-operative management

After cataract extraction, the eye will be without its lens. Therefore an intraocular lens has to be inserted or cataract glasses have to be used in order that objects can be focused sharply on the retina. Unfortunately, the thick cataract glasses usually with a dioptric power of +10 tends to lead to difficulty in adjustment owing to the enlarged image size, the peripheral distortion, and the image jump. The use of contact lenses minimise the problem. But older patients usually find contact lenses difficult to manage. An intraocular lens placed within the eyeball at the time of surgery gives excellent post-operative vision. It is now the procedure of choice.

Secondary cataract

Secondary cataract can develop in association with other diseases of the eye such as following iridocyclitis or retinal detachment. It is sometimes associated with trauma from injury or surgery.

GLAUCOMA

In the normal eye, there is a delicate balance between the inflow and outflow of aqueous. When the outflow is blocked, the intraocular pressure rises, leading to optic nerve damage. This condition is known as glaucoma.

There are two main types of glaucoma:
- Open-angle glaucoma which develops insidiously and leads to visual loss with few or no symptoms.
- Closed-angle glaucoma which develops suddenly is associated with acute pain, sudden visual loss and congestion of the eye. Because of the congestion, acute closed-angle glaucoma frequently presents as a unilateral red eye.

Open-angle glaucoma is more common than closed-angle glaucoma among Caucasians while closed-angle glaucoma is more common among the Chinese. Glaucoma causes 10% of blindness in most countries.

CHRONIC OPEN-ANGLE GLAUCOMA

Chronic open-angle glaucoma is a condition of raised intraocular pressure associated with visual loss. Although the filtration angle is open, the trabecular meshwork at the filtration angle is defective, leading to increased resistance to the outflow of aqueous.

The diagnosis is confirmed by a combination of raised intraocular pressure, visual field loss and glaucomatous cupping of the optic disc. It is an insidious condition usually presenting with no symptoms. The symptoms, if present, are not dramatic and consist of frequent changes of glasses, vague tiredness, ocular discomfort and increased difficulty with reading.

Ocular hypertension

An intraocular pressure of more than 20 mm Hg suggests the possibility of glaucoma. It is useful to note that a number of patients with raised intraocular pressure of 30 mm Hg do not suffer any visual loss. This condition is called "ocular hypertension" and usually requires no treatment, except careful and regular reviews.

Visual field loss

Typical visual field changes develop in chronic open-angle glaucoma. Early changes include an arcuate scotoma and later, the loss of the nasal field. Late changes leave the patient with restricted central vision although sometimes some temporal vision remains.

Optic cup

There is usually an increase in size of the optic disc cup in association with the visual field loss. In advanced chronic open-angle glaucoma, the cup reaches the edge of the disc. The retinal vessels dip sharply over the edge of the cup and there is optic atrophy.

Cup/disc ratio

As the size of the normal physiological cup varies with different individuals it can be difficult to distinguish a glaucomatous cup from a physiological cup. A method used to record the size of the optic disc cup is the cup/disc ratio. If the cup reaches the margins of the disc, it is designated 1.0. If the cup extends across 40% of the disc diameter, it is recorded as 0.4. If the cup/disc ratio is greater than 0.5 or if there is asymmetry, the possibility of glaucoma should be excluded.

Prevention and early diagnosis

Diagnosis is frequently made too late because of the lack of symptoms in chronic open-angle glaucoma. To prevent this, periodic measurement of intraocular pressure in all patients over the age of 40 is advisable as open-angle glaucoma has been found in 1%-2% of older patients in many countries.

There is also a familial tendency in this condition. All relatives of patients with chronic open-angle glaucoma should be regularly reviewed.

Treatment is usually medical. The therapy of choice is Pilocarpine 4 times a day or Timolol 0.25%-0.5% twice a day. Additional drugs include 1%-2% Adrenalin, Propine 1% and oral Acetazolamide. If medical therapy proves unsatisfactory then laser trabeculoplasty may be used. This is effective in the majority of cases. But if it is not effective then microsurgical trabeculectomy should be considered.

ACUTE CLOSED-ANGLE GLAUCOMA

Acute closed-angle glaucoma is common in middle-aged patients. Any middle-aged patient with a unilateral red eye associated with blurred vision, pain or headache, should be suspected of having acute closed-angle glaucoma. It occurs when the iris periphery suddenly apposes itself to the corneal periphery and blocks the filtration angle. This prevents aqueous from flowing into the outflow channel, leading to a sudden rise in intraocular pressure.

The patient is frequently in pain, the eye is congested, and the cornea is hazy due to epithelial oedema which is the initial cause of the blurred vision. The pupil is semi-dilated and not reactive to light. The anterior chamber is shallow but this is not easily observed. If this is unrelieved, the increased pressure will cause permanent damage to the eye, resulting in severe visual loss or blindness.

Treatment is urgent. The patient should be referred to an ophthalmologist as soon as possible. Surgery is required after the intraocular pressure has been medically reduced.

Medical therapy

Immediate intensive medical therapy to lower the intraocular pressure is important. 1%-4% Pilocarpine should be instilled every ten minutes for the first hour, then less frequently. Acetazolamide (500 mg) should be administered intravenously. Oral Acetazolamide (1000 mg) should be given and repeated every four hours. Osmotic agents such as Glycerol or intravenous Mannitol may be used. An analgesic or tranquilliser should be given where appropriate. Treatment must continue until the pressure is reduced.

Surgery

Peripheral iridectomy is the treatment of choice. It is simple and safe. Alternatively, a minute iridotomy can be done with either the argon or neodynium YAG laser. However, a filtration operation may be necessary especially for patients who have failed to respond to medical therapy. The decision on the type of surgery to be performed and the timing for it can be determined only after careful evaluation of the patient's condition by an ophthalmologist.

The fellow eye

Acute closed-angle glaucoma is bilateral. The fellow eye is at risk of developing an acute attack in 50% of cases in five years. A prophylactic peripheral iridectomy should be performed on the fellow eye. More recently, laser iridotomy has been used successfully.

Subacute and chronic closed-angle glaucoma

When the filtration angle is less rapidly closed, the rise of pressure will be subacute (subacute glaucoma). Accordingly, the symptoms will be milder. The patient may complain of having transient blurred vision, mild headache and of seeing 'halos' (rainbow colours around lights). Closed-angle glaucoma may even simulate chronic open-angle glaucoma and has no symptoms until there is severe visual field loss at an advanced stage of the condition (chronic closed-angle glaucoma). Diagnosis for chronic closed-angle glaucoma is made by gonioscopy.

SECONDARY GLAUCOMA

The intraocular pressure may be increased by a disease process which blocks the outflow channel of the aqueous. In severe iridocyclitis, the inflammatory proteins and cells or iris adhesions may block up the outflow channel. In hyphaema, (blood in the anterior chamber), the outflow channel may be blocked by the blood. New iris vessels which may develop with central retinal vein occlusion and proliferative diabetic retinopathy may lead to secondary haemorrhagic glaucoma which is difficult to treat. Sometimes, glaucoma is a complication of a mature cataract or intraocular tumours.

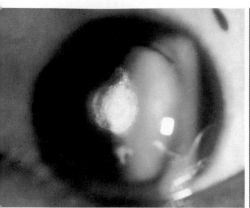

Fig. 4.1
Central cortical cataract. Vision worse in bright sunlight or while reading when pupil constricts.

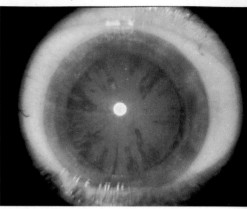

Fig. 4.2
Peripheral cortical cataract. Vision usually affected later.

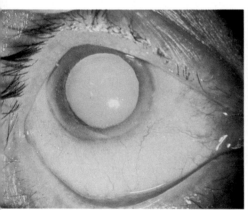

Fig. 4.3
Mature cataract where entire lens becomes opaque. Maturity can lead to complications.

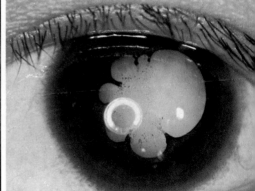

Fig. 4.4
Cataract secondary to iridocyclitis. Note adhesions between iris and anterior lens capsule (posterior synechia).

Visual Field Loss in Open-angle Glaucoma

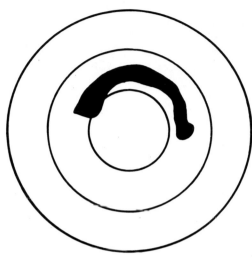

Fig. 4.5
Arcuate scotoma in early glaucoma.

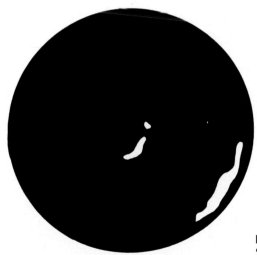

Fig. 4.6
Severe visual field loss in advanced glaucoma.

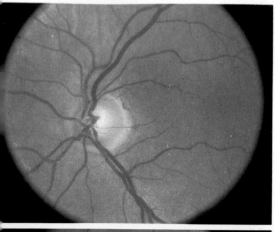

Fig. 4.7
Normal optic disc with cup/disc ratio 0.4.

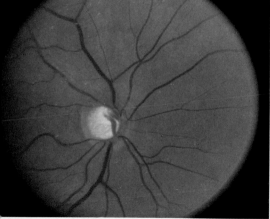

Fig. 4.8
Glaucomatous cup with cup/disc ratio 0.7 and early visual field defect.

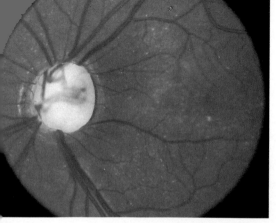

Fig. 4.9
Large terminal glaucomatous cup with cup/disc ratio 1.0 and optic atrophy (note: eye is blind).

Closed-angle Glaucoma

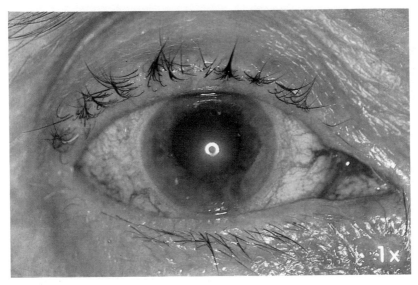

Fig. 4.10
Acute congestive closed-angle glaucoma. Seen as red eye with hazy cornea and fixed dilated pupil.

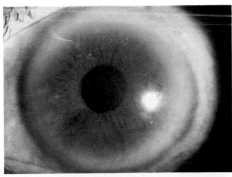

Fig. 4.11
Peripheral iridectomy — operation of choice in closed-angle glaucoma.

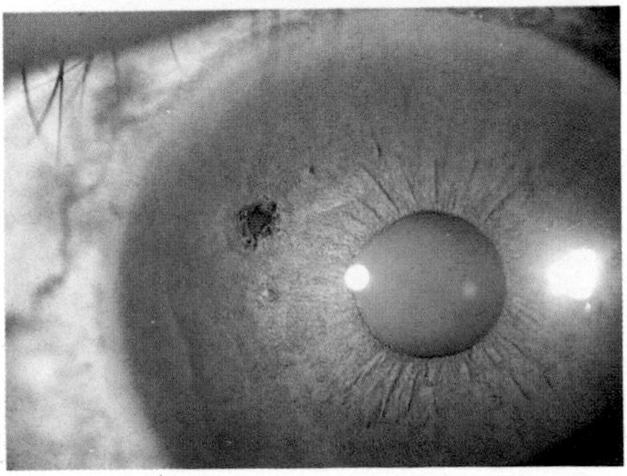

Fig. 4.12
Laser iridotomy.

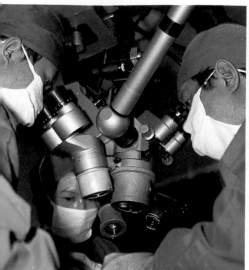

Fig. 4.13
Operating microscope – now used by most ophthalmic surgeons for all anterior segment operations.

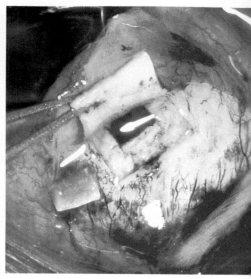

Fig. 4.14
Trabeculectomy, a commonly used filtrating operation for glaucoma.

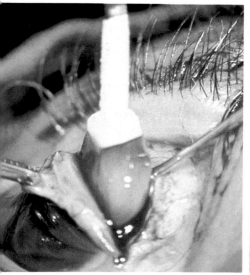

Fig. 4.15
Intracapsular cataract extraction with cryopencil.

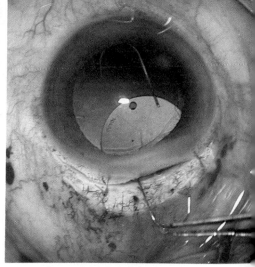

Fig. 4.16
Microscopic extracapsular cataract extraction with posterior chamber lens is method of choice in many countries.

5

UVEAL TRACT, RETINA AND VITREOUS

INTRODUCTION

Inflammation of the uvea (uveitis) is sometimes related to systemic disease. Similarly, various retinal vascular conditions, including retinal artery and vein occlusions are associated with cardiovascular diseases.

Retinal detachment is a cause of sudden painless visual loss. It should be referred for urgent surgery. With modern surgical techniques, the prognosis is good.

Pathologic macular conditions are important. More than half of recent blindness in developed countries is due to diseases affecting the macula. Of particular importance are age-related macular degeneration, high myopia and diabetic retinopathy.

UVEITIS

Iridocyclitis (iritis)

Iridocyclitis, the inflammation of the iris and ciliary body, usually presents as a painful unilateral red eye. It must be differentiated from other common causes of a unilateral red eye, including acute closed-angle glaucoma, foreign body injury, keratitis and corneal ulcer.

The symptoms include photophobia, mild pain, blurred vision and watering. The pupil is small and slit-lamp examination shows flare (proteins) and cells in the anterior chamber as well as deposits of white cells (keratic precipitates) on the posterior surface of the cornea. The inflamed iris may adhere to the anterior capsule of the lens (posterior synechia). When the iridocyclitis is severe, secondary glaucoma and secondary cataract may result. This condition tends to recur.

The cause is usually difficult to determine. It may be associated with joint diseases such as ankylosing spondylitis or Still's disease (juvenile rheumatoid arthritis) but rarely with sarcoidosis, syphilis, leprosy, tuberculosis or viral infection.

Cycloplegics such as Atropine or Homatropine are used to dilate the pupil and prevent posterior synechia. They also relieve the pain. Steroid eyedrops reduce the inflammation. Investigations should be carried out to exclude the known causes in severe and recurrent iridocyclitis.

Chorioretinitis

Inflammation of the choroid and the retina, chorioretinitis, usually presents with visual loss.

In the acute stage, if the inflammation is at the macula, the patient will present with visual loss. Lesions which are not at the macula may be silent and are found only when routine examination shows a chorioretinal scar. In pars planitis (chorioretinitis at the extreme fundal periphery), the condition may remain silent for many months or years and it only manifests itself when the vision is affected by vitreous opacities or macular oedema.

In the majority the cause is unknown. In some cases, it may be due to toxoplasmosis. Less commonly, it is associated with syphilis, tuberculosis, sarcoidosis, toxocara (worms) and histoplasmosis.

Investigations to find the cause should be carried out. Treatment can be difficult. The use of systemic steroid may help in addition to therapy for specific infections. Recurrences are common.

CHOROIDAL TUMOUR

Naevus (benign choroidal melanoma)

A naevus is a flat, round, pigmented, choroidal lesion rarely causing any visual disturbance. It is usually easy to distinguish between a flat benign naevus and a raised malignant choroidal melanoma.

Malignant choroidal melanoma

A pigmented, raised lesion of the choroid is usually a malignant choroidal melanoma. It sometimes presents with retinal detachment, and occasionally with vitreous haemorrhage or secondary glaucoma. Because of this, malignant melanoma should be excluded in unilateral blind eyes of uncertain etiology. It is more common in Caucasians than in other races.

Enucleation of the eye is usually required. In selected patients with only one good eye left, or those with small tumours, irradiation, photocoagulation or surgical excision may be used. Recent statistics indicate that small, malignant choroidal melanoma may be kept under observation but without treatment, provided they are regularly evaluated.

Choroidal metastasis

Choroidal metastasis may result from a wide variety of cancers including breast and lung cancer. It is rare. It usually presents in the eye as flat multiple deposits at the posterior pole. Usually it is associated with an exudative retinal detachment. Treatment with radiotherapy may help to retain vision for the limited lifespan of the patient.

VASCULAR OCCLUSION

Central retinal artery occlusion

In occlusion of the central retinal artery the patient notices sudden visual loss in one eye and, within a few minutes, the eye may become totally blind.

Complete obstruction of the central retinal artery presents a characteristic ophthalmoscopic picture a few hours after the attack. The larger retinal arteries are constricted and look like thin threads while the smaller vessels are scarcely visible. The fundus appears milky white because of retinal oedema. In contrast to this, there is a cherry-red spot at the macula where the retina is thin and where the red choroidal circulation shows through. Haemorrhages are not seen in central retinal artery occlusion unless the vein is also occluded.

After a few weeks, the retinal swelling subsides and the retina regains its transparency but the disc becomes pale because of atrophy of the optic nerve. The retinal arterioles remain narrow.

The use of vasodilators and emergency attempts to lower the intraocular pressure are normally ineffective. However, if treatment is given within a few hours of the onset, there is a slight chance of visual recovery. For this reason, treatment should be attempted. Elderly patients with central retinal artery occlusion must exclude temporal arteritis by blood ESR and occasionally, by biopsy of the temporal artery. Failure to recognise this cause, which is controlled with high doses of steroids, may lead to blindness in the fellow eye.

The more common causes of central retinal artery occlusion include arteriosclerosis with or without hypertension and emboli from diseased heart valves or carotid atheroma.

Central retinal vein occlusion

Occlusion of the central retinal vein is less abrupt in presentation than occlusion of the central retinal artery. Visual impairment occurs gradually and the loss of sight is less complete. The patient is left with visual acuity of counting fingers.

The predisposing causes are hypertension, diabetes mellitus, arteriosclerosis in the elderly, open-angle glaucoma and factors or conditions which increase coagulability of the blood including the use of oral contraceptives.

Examination with the ophthalmoscope shows grossly tortuous and engorged retinal veins, especially near the optic disc. Very often, unilateral disc oedema is present. Scattered all over the retina, from the disc to the periphery, are haemorrhages of all shapes and sizes. These are accompanied by soft exudates.

After a period of many weeks, the haemorrhages clear gradually and there is little evidence of the occlusion, except for shunt vessels on the optic disc. Vision fails to be restored in the majority of the elderly but the prognosis for younger patients is better.

The development of new vessels on the iris (rubeosis iridis) is due to ischaemia of the retina. These vessels may obstruct drainage in the filtration angle and cause painful secondary thrombotic glaucoma. This happens in about one-third of the patients if untreated with laser.

Medical investigations may reveal predisposing systemic diseases. Photocoagulation is used to prevent secondary thrombotic glaucoma. If this condition develops, medical therapy to lower the pressure may control the pain.

Branch retinal vein occlusion

The visual symptoms depend on the site of occlusion. If the macula is involved, the patient will complain of blurred vision. The fundal changes show a characteristic fan-shaped distribution of retinal haemorrhages which radiate from the arteriovenous crossings. The haemorrhages are usually flame-shaped.

Macular oedema may sometimes persist, and swelling disrupt the fovea leading to visual loss. Moreover, vitreous haemorrhage from abnormal retinal vessels, either shunt or new vessels, may cause sudden visual loss.

After some months, there is re-establishment of local circulation around the site of the occlusion and the haemorrhages and exudates are absorbed.

Branch retinal vein occlusion usually occurs at an arterovenous junction, that is, where a vein is crossed by a sclerotic artery. The superior temporal vein is the branch most commonly affected. If either this vein or the inferior temporal vein is occluded, the macula may be involved. The main predisposing causes of branch retinal vein occlusion are longstanding hypertension (85%), arteriosclerosis and diabetes.

Laser photocoagulation may be used to ablate the damaged capillary bed if macular oedema decreases vision or when there is danger of vitreous haemorrhage from abnormal new vessels.

RETINAL DETACHMENT

Retinal detachment is caused by tears (holes) which are usually located at the peripheral areas of the retina. These tears develop in degenerate or thin retina. An important factor is degenerate vitreous which collapses with age and may cause traction. Retinal detachment is most common in patients with degenerative (high) myopia, in the elderly and as a result of ocular injuries.

The symptoms of a retinal tear include seeing multiple floaters of recent onset and flashes of light. Vitreous floaters have been described by patients as dots, flies or cobwebs in their field of vision. Even if the patient has seen single floaters for many months, it is usually harmless.

On the other hand, a large number of floaters appearing suddenly together with flashes of light in patients with myopia or in the elderly requires retinal assessment by an ophthalmologist. Retinal tears may cause vitreous haemorrhage or lead to separation of the retina from the pigment epithelium and choroid, resulting in sudden visual loss.

With the development of retinal detachment there is in addition loss of peripheral visual field. The typical symptom described is "a curtain obstructing part of the vision". If the macula is affected, there is a sudden loss of central vision.

Ophthalmoscopy shows a loss of the red reflex with areas of detached retina appearing grey and undulating.

A superior temporal detachment is an ocular emergency. The spread of the subretinal fluid due to gravity may detach the macula leading to permanent defective central vision. Bed rest is urgently required until surgery can be carried out.

Diagnosis is confirmed by an ophthalmologist by examining the retina with full dilatation of the pupils with an indirect ophthalmoscope. The indirect ophthalmoscope gives a better view of the peripheral retina than the direct ophthalmoscope.

It is important to find all the retinal tears (holes) as all the tears have to be sealed with firm scars. These scars are produced by cryoapplication, diathermy or photocoagulation. For technical reasons, cryoapplication is the most popular. Silicone is sometimes used to push the wall of the sclera inwards to close the tear.

As retinal detachment is a bilateral disease, similar changes are frequently found in the other eye which should also be thoroughly examined with the indirect ophthalmoscope.

Exudative and traction retinal detachment

Less commonly, retinal detachment is not due to a retinal tear but exudation as in malignant choroidal melanoma, severe uveitis or toxaemia of pregnancy. Another cause of detachment is fibrous traction in proliferative diabetic retinopathy or retrolental fibroplasia.

MACULAR DISEASES

Macular diseases are major causes of blindness. In developed countries, blindness today is rarely caused by infection or malnutrition but mainly by degenerative, metabolic and vascular conditions affecting the macula.

Local macular lesions which cause gradual loss of central vision include degenerative high myopia, juvenile macular dystrophy and age-related macular degeneration. The common acute macular conditions are central serous retinopathy, macular haemorrhages, and disciform macular degeneration. Diffuse retinal conditions which affect the macula include retinal vein occlusion and diabetic retinopathy.

Many macular diseases are as yet untreatable. More effective treatment can be developed only with a better understanding of retinal metabolism and pathophysiology.

Juvenile macular dystrophy

This occurs in the young who often has a history of a similar disease in the family. It is bilateral and symmetrical and causes gradual painless loss of vision. A variety of clinical entities exist with presumably different underlying genetic defects.

There is no effective treatment. Precise diagnosis, visual aids and genetic and occupational counselling are useful.

Age-related maculopathy

Age-related maculopathy (senile macular degeneration) is a bilateral degeneration of the macula. It causes loss of central vision. It accounts for over 20% of blindness in Caucasians (less than 6/60 visual acuity) but is less prevalent in other races.

The patient usually complains of gradual increasing disturbance of central vision. One letter or word may appear at a different level from its neighbour or there may be missing letters or words.

The ophthalmoscopic picture varies. The macula usually has fine pigmentary clumps and patches of atrophy. White round spots called drusen (colloid bodies) are frequently seen. If large or confluent, the drusen is frequently associated with macular degeneration. If fine and sharply-demarcated, the drusen is usually harmless.

Disciform degeneration of the macula

Sometimes, vision may be suddenly lost because of an acute complication of age-related maculopathy. A localised, raised exudative lesion which is usually disciform in shape develops at the macula. This is usually associated with new vessel proliferation from the choroid (subretinal neovascularisation).

Urgent fundal fluorescein angiographic tests should be carried out, as subretinal neovascularisation at an early stage may be effectively treated with laser photocoagulation.

It is important to emphasize to patients with macular degeneration that they will not go totally blind from the condition as peripheral vision will not be affected. Some patients benefit from the use of strong glasses and a variety of visual aids for distant and near vision. These include magnifying lenses and special telescopic spectacles.

Central serous retinopathy

This condition is common in males from 20 to 50 years of age. It occurs spontaneously and is characterised by fluid leaking from the choroidal capillaries through the pigment epithelium and subsequently accumulating under the macula. The etiology is unknown.

The patient complains of sudden disturbance of central vision which is generally described as a dulling, darkening or blurring of vision. In most cases, there is micropsia (objects appearing smaller) and the ability to discriminate colour is sometimes reduced.

Ophthalmoscopically, the macula shows a characteristic round swelling with a ring reflex at its border. Diagnosis is confirmed by fundal fluorescein angiography which shows a leaking defect in the retinal pigment epithelium.

The condition is usually self-limiting and benign. If severe or if it persists for many months, photocoagulation may be used. Recurrences are common.

Degenerative (high) myopia

Degenerative myopia is often familial and is characterised by a progressive increase in the axial length of the eye and by chorioretinal atrophy. The atrophy is more pronounced at the posterior pole of the eye and may cause loss of central vision, sometimes from macular haemorrhage. The loss of central vision is proportional to the amount of macular involvement. Another complication which may develop is detachment of the retina.

Direct ophthalmoscopy is difficult owing to the high refractive error. The view is improved by examining the fundus through the patient's glasses or contact lenses. The disc shows a typical crescent or ring of chorioretinal atrophy surrounding its margin.

No treatment can change the progress of this condition. Vocational guidance may be useful prior to the loss of central vision. The rate of deterioration is unpredictable.

Retinitis pigmentosa

Retinitis pigmentosa is characterised by defective vision in dim light and progressive loss of peripheral field. The hereditary pattern may be recessive, dominant or sex-linked. Onset of symptoms is in the first or second decade of life. The vision usually deteriorates to blindness by the fifth or sixth decade. The ophthalmoscopic signs include proliferation of retinal pigment with a characteristic dark brown spider-like appearance, a waxy-yellow disc and attenuated retinal vessels.

It is important to study the family history in this condition to establish genetic risks. Electroretinography is abnormal before ophthalmoscopic signs develop.

Retinitis pigmentosa is sometimes associated with a variety of rare systemic abnormalities such as deafness, cataract and glaucoma. Therefore, regular ophthalmic examination is recommended.

VITREOUS CONDITIONS

Degeneration of the vitreous occurs as a result of age and in high myopia. The vitreous becomes more fluid and may spontaneously detached itself from the retina. As it causes flashes and floaters, the presence of a retinal tear has to be excluded. Floaters are a particularly common ocular complaint and are usually harmless.

Other forms of vitreal degeneration which are sometimes present but harmless are white deposits, asteroid bodies and synchisis scintillans.

Vitreous haemorrhage is a cause of sudden visual loss. It is caused by trauma, retinal tear or abnormal blood vessels, especially in diabetic retinopathy. The blood may be absorbed over many months. However, if the blood does not absorb, vitrectomy — a surgical method of removing blood from the vitreous — may help to restore vision in blind eyes.

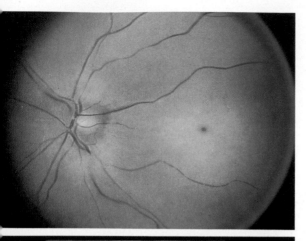

Fig. 5.1
Typical central retinal artery occlusion showing cherry-red spot surrounded by white retinal oedema. Retinal vessels are narrow. Eye is blind.

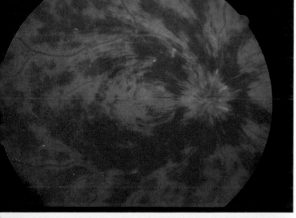

Fig. 5.2
Central retinal vein occlusion showing multiple flame-shaped haemorrhages, soft exudates and optic disc oedema.

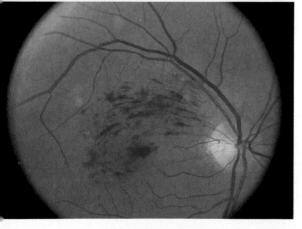

Fig. 5.3
Branch occlusion of superior temporal retinal vein causing flame-shaped retinal haemorrhages.

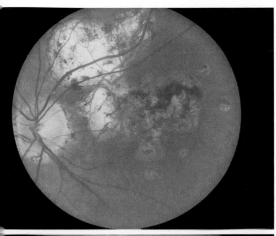

Fig. 5.4
Disseminated pigmented chorioretinal scars following non-specific chorioretinitis.

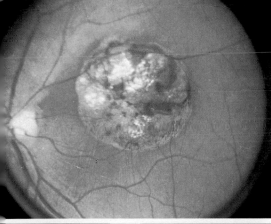

Fig. 5.5
Macular pigmented chorioretinal scar from presumed toxoplasmosis..

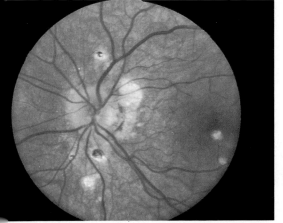

Fig. 5.6
Small, round, pigmented chorioretinal scars from presumed histoplasmosis.

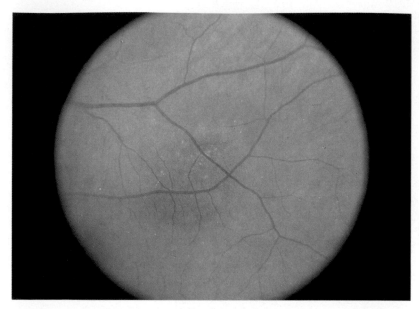

Fig. 5.7
Benign naevus choroidal melanoma – pigmented, flat and stationary.

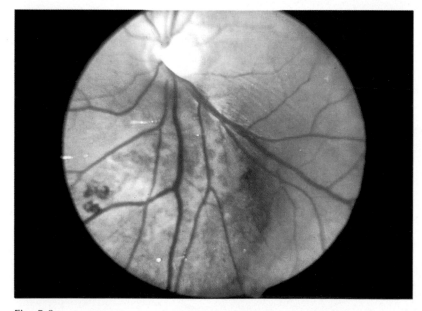

Fig. 5.8
Malignant melanoma of choroid – pigmented, raised and enlarging.

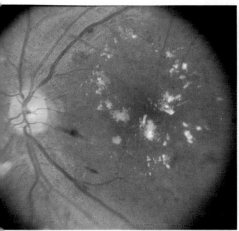

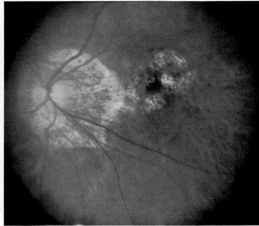

Fig. 5.9
Maculopathy of diabetic retinopathy with exudates and oedema of macula.

Fig. 5.10
Pigmented macular chorioretinal atrophy of degenerative (high) myopia. Note atrophy around optic disc.

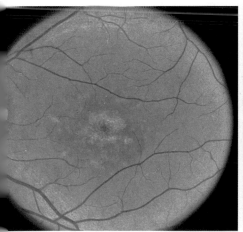

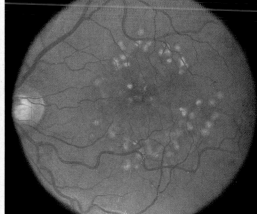

Fig. 5.11
Juvenile hereditary macular dystrophy.

Fig. 5.12
Drusen (colloid bodies) of macula with good visual acuity.

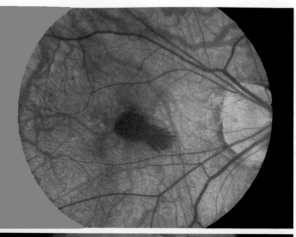

Fig. 5.13
Macular haemorrhage in degenerate (high) myopia. (Note visible choroidal vessels and atrophy around optic disc).

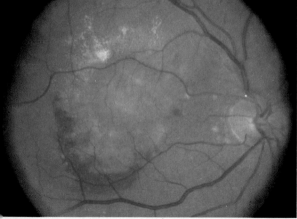

Fig. 5.14
Disciform macular degeneration of old age with subretinal fluid, exudates and haemorrhage.

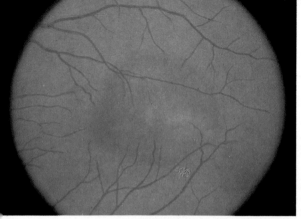

Fig. 5.15
Central serous retinopathy with localised subretinal fluid at macula.

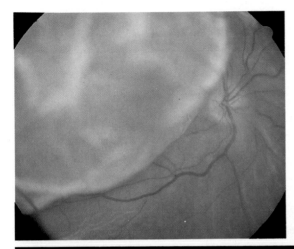

Fig. 5.16
Ballooning superior temporal retinal detachment. (Note detachment has spread to involve almost entire retina.)

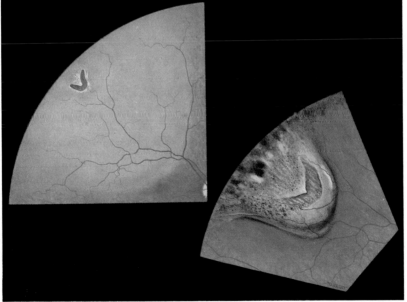

Fig. 5.17
Retinal detachment due to retinal tear (above). Tear sealed by freezing and silicone buckle (below).

(Courtesy of the Institute of Ophthalmology, London)

6

OCULAR MANIFESTATIONS OF SYSTEMIC DISEASES

INTRODUCTION

Many systemic diseases have ocular manifestations. The most important is diabetic retinopathy. Laser photocoagulation prevents blindness in the majority of patients if treatment is started early.

Other systemic conditions affecting the eye are hypertension, thyroid and rheumatoid diseases. In some developing countries, keratomalacia (Vitamin A deficiency) and onchocerciasis (filarial worm infection) are major causes of blindness.

DIABETES MELLITUS

Refractive changes

Blurring of vision in a diabetic patient is sometimes the result of refractive changes in the eye. These are due to fluctuation in the blood-sugar level and occur frequently when diabetics commence treatment. The patient should be assured that the refractive changes will stop once the blood-sugar level is stabilised and that the condition will not cause any permanent loss of vision.

Extraocular muscle paralysis

Diabetes sometimes affects the third or sixth cranial nerve. A third cranial nerve lesion due to diabetes may be associated with a unilateral headache. The pupil is usually not affected. The condition resolves itself within three months.

Pupil and iris abnormalities

The pupils may respond sluggishly to light or fail to dilate with mydriatic eyedrops. Neovascularisation of the iris may develop (rubeosis iridis) in some patients with severe proliferative diabetic retinopathy.

Cataract

Senile cataract develops more often in a diabetic and at a younger age. It may develop rapidly as a dense fluffy white cataract in a young diabetic with severe uncontrolled diabetes.

DIABETIC RETINOPATHY

The most important ocular manifestation of diabetes is diabetic retinopathy. It is now a major cause of blindness in developed countries and is rapidly becoming an important cause of blindness in some developing countries.

The development of diabetic retinopathy is related to the length of time that the patient has had diabetes. The main reason for the increase in diabetic retinopathy in recent years is that with better medical treatment diabetics now live longer. In some countries diabetic retinopathy has been found in one third of the diabetic population.

Classification of diabetic retinopathy

(1) Background diabetic retinopathy
(2) Proliferative diabetic retinopathy

(1) BACKGROUND DIABETIC RETINOPATHY

The changes are usually found at the posterior pole, in the area between the superior temporal and the inferior temporal retinal vessels. They consist of retinal microaneurysms, round dot haemorrhages and hard exudates. The characteristic minute red round spots are either micro-aneurysms or dot haemorrhages. The hard exudates appear as minute yellow, well-defined deposits. These are usually multiple and scattered. They may become more extensive later and form large confluent patches.

With maculopathy

Background diabetic retinopathy progresses slowly over the years. The majority of the patients do not lose their central vision. Some develop changes in the macula resulting in the deterioration of central vision. This complication of diabetic retinopathy is known as maculopathy. Depending on the amount of haemorrhage and exudate, the degree of oedema and capillary loss at the macula, the vision can fall to less than 6/60 in severe maculopathy.

(2) PROLIFERATIVE DIABETIC RETINOPATHY

Vascular obstructive changes are seen in pre-proliferative diabetic retinopathy. These obstructive features include soft exudates (cotton wool spots), large blot haemorrhages, dilated or segmented veins and venous loops. These changes indicate more severe (ischaemic) retinal damage. Fundal fluorescein angiography shows loss of capillary circulation.

Neovascularisation develops in about 10% of patients with diabetic retinopathy. The new vessels grow on the retinal surface and at the optic disc. They tend to bleed into the vitreous. Fibrous tissue formation leads to traction retinal detachment.

Prognosis

The visual prognosis depends on the type and severity of the retinopathy. Most patients with background diabetic retinopathy do not develop visual loss. In proliferative diabetic retinopathy, the visual outlook is worse. The presence of diabetic retinopathy, especially proliferative diabetic retinopathy, usually reflects the general state of health of the patient. Renal and microvascular complications may result in a shorter life span.

Management

If laser photocoagulation is done at an early stage, the majority of blindness from diabetic retinopathy is preventable.

As the early fundal changes can be easily missed, the fundus of all diabetics should be regularly examined with the pupils dilated.

All diabetics without fundal changes require strict metabolic control and dietary advice to delay or prevent the development of diabetic retinopathy and other complications. The patients should have annual fundal examination to detect early retinal changes.

Diabetics with retinopathy require an analysis of their diet, metabolic control and life-style. The presence of retinopathy should be regarded as a warning that the control may have been sub-optimal over an extended period of time. Ophthalmic assessment should include colour fundal photography and fundal fluorescein angiography. If vision is threatened, photocoagulation should be carried out.

Photocoagulation

A photocoagulator produces intense light (argon laser or xenon) which is focused on the retinal pigment epithelium where the light beam is converted to heat. The resulting small chorioretinal burns form scars and destroy abnormal vessels.

Photocoagulation is effective in preventing blindness due to diabetic retinopathy. It should be carried out in the presence of diabetic maculopathy or pre-proliferative diabetic retinopathy. In proliferative diabetic retinopathy, extensive photocoagulation (known as pan retinal photocoagulation) is necessary to prevent vitreous haemorrhage and traction retinal detachment.

HYPERTENSION AND ARTERIOSCLEROSIS

Hypertension primarily affects the retinal arterioles. In young patients the arterioles react to moderately raised blood pressure by constriction. The ophthalmic signs are either diffuse or focal constriction of the arterioles.

In middle-aged patients however, the walls of the arterioles become thickened (arteriosclerosis) and are unable to constrict. The thickened walls show a widening of the normal light reflex. As the thickening of the wall progresses, it gives a copper appearance to the blood column (copper wiring) and then a white appearance (silver wiring). At the arteriovenous crossings, the thickened arteriolar walls displace and constrict the veins (arteriovenous nipping). These changes are common in middle-aged patients with chronic hypertension. They may lead to a branch retinal vein occlusion.

In more severe hypertensives, the arteriolar wall is damaged by necrosis leading to flame-shaped haemorrhages and soft exudates (cotton wool spots) caused by microinfarcts of the retina. Sometimes retinal oedema is present. Chronic retinal oedema at the macula results in hard exudates radiating from the macula (macular star). Finally papilloedema results. When this happens, the patient has malignant hypertension. Vision is usually normal except when there is associated macular involvement.

Hypertensive retinopathy

Many attempts have been made to classify hypertensive retinopathy, of which the Keith-Wagner classification is the most useful. In the first two grades changes are limited to the retinal vessels, but in Grade III, retinal haemorrhages and soft exudates are present. In Grade IV there is papilloedema.

Grade I

In young patients with mild hypertension, minimum constriction and irregularity of the arterioles are found. In older hypertensives however, there is often no arteriolar constriction but a widening of the light reflex of the arterioles because of the thickened sclerotic arteriolar wall.

Grade II

The arteriolar changes in Grade II are similar to those of Grade I except that they are more obvious. The retinal veins at the arteriovenous crossings appear constricted and are seen ophthalmoscopically as arteriovenous nippings.

Grade III

Superficial flame-shaped haemorrhages appear near the disc with soft exudates. The retina is oedematous. Occasionally, small hard exudates may also appear.

Grade IV

Papilloedema is an ominous sign of malignant hypertension. When retinal oedema is substantial and prolonged, small hard exudates collect and radiate from the macula in a characteristic star-shaped formation.

Significance

The significance of grading is that the fundal changes reflect the severity of the hypertension and the state of the arterioles elsewhere in the body. Furthermore, when the fundal changes are reversed, it serves as a good indication of the control of the hypertension.

Pre-eclamptic hypertension

In pre-eclamptic toxaemia or hypertension of pregnancy, there is a marked spasm of the arterioles as they are not sclerotic in young patients. All the more severe signs of hypertension may be superimposed. The condition is frequently associated with bilateral exudative inferior retinal detachment.

Other vascular retinopathies

Severe anaemia is frequently associated with flame-shaped haemorrhages and soft exudates. The retinopathy has no unique features and is common in conditions where there is an associated platelet deficiency such as in penicious anaemia and leukaemia.

Hyperviscosity retinopathy occurs in any condition which increases the blood viscosity such as hyperglobulinaemia and polycythaemia vera. The retinal veins are engorged, associated with retinal haemorrhages, occasional soft exudates and oedema. The fundus is very similar to that found in central retinal vein occlusion.

Sickle-cell anaemia is a hereditary condition (ss or sc haemoglobin) common in Negroid populations. Owing to occlusion of small vessels at the retinal periphery and ischaemia, fibrovascular proliferation occurs. Localised chorioretinal scars are also characteristic of the condition. Vision may be lost from vitreous haemorrhage or traction retinal detachment but this can be prevented with photocoagulation.

Peripheral retinal vasculitis with vitreous haemorrhage (Eales' disease) is characterised by recurrent vitreous haemorrhages associated with abnormalities of the peripheral retinal veins. This condition occurs particularly in young adult males who are otherwise well. The cause is unknown but was once thought to be due to sensitisation to tuberculosis. Photocoagulation or cryotherapy of abnormal retinal vessels can prevent recurrent vitreous haemorrhage. Blindness from vitreous haemorrhage can be reversed in many cases by vitrectomy.

THYROID DISEASE

Hyperthyroidism (Graves' disease)

Hyperthyroidism is associated with lid retraction and lid lag, and sometimes, with exophthalmos. The eyelid signs may be unilateral or bilateral. Bilateral lid retraction gives a typical staring appearance. Other signs include poor convergence and infrequent blinking.

Thyroid exophthalmos

Thyroid exophthalmos is caused by orbital oedema and lymphocyte infiltration. It may develop with or without hyperthyroidism, or following treatment for hyperthyroidism. The ocular signs are exophthalmos with oedema of the lids and conjunctiva. Sometimes there is restriction of ocular movement, particularly for elevation. As a result, the patient is unable to look upwards. Although the exophthalmos is usually bilateral it can be unilateral. A CT scan is useful for diagnosis. It helps to differentiate a unilateral exophthalmos from that of a retrobulbar space-occupying lesion and it usually shows typical thickened extraocular muscles.

Complications

Severe thyroid exophthalmos may lead to difficulty in closing the eyelids, a condition known as lagophthalmos. This may cause exposure keratitis with corneal dryness, ulceration and infection. The increased intraorbital pressure may also damage the optic nerve.

Treatment

Hyperthyroidism should be treated. High doses of oral steroids may control the progressive exophthalmos. Surgery may be necessary to protect the cornea or to decompress the orbit. Surgical correction of diplopia after the disease has burnt itself out may also be necessary.

INFECTION AND MALNUTRITION

In developing countries, infections and nutritional diseases like onchocerciasis and keratomalacia are major causes of blindness. Their eradication depends on dealing with the problems of poverty — poor living conditions, diet and health education at grass root level with the help of thousands of paramedics. In the People's Republic of China, the "barefoot" doctors are reported to be effective in controlling blindness which has resulted from malnutrition and infection.

Keratomalacia (Vitamin A deficiency)

Keratomalacia is an acute condition of the cornea due to Vitamin A deficiency in the child. It is frequently precipitated by a gastrointestinal upset. It starts with xerosis (dryness of the conjunctiva) and may lead to melting and perforation of the cornea (keratomalacia). The International Agency for the Prevention of Blindness has estimated that a quarter of a million children in the world are blinded annually by this condition.

Onchocerciasis (river blindness)

This major blinding condition is due to the invasion by microfilariae resulting from the bite of the jinja-fly which is common in parts of West Africa. The eye complications include iritis, secondary glaucoma, cataract and vitreoretinal damage. Blindness is common in the affected communities. The condition is prevented by the elimination of the vector fly. This is unfortunately not always possible. Treatment of the established condition with antihelminthic drugs or surgery does not restore vision.

Leprosy

This affects the eye in 30% of the cases but most of the ocular complications are not serious. The facial nerve may be involved resulting in paralysis of the orbicularis oculi muscle, ectropion (everted lid) and lagophthalmos (inability to close the lids) leading to exposure keratitis. There may also be madarosis (loss of eyebrows and eyelashes). Keratitis and anterior uveitis are uncommon.

Syphilis

This may affect the eye at all stages of the disease. The primary sore rarely occurs on the eyelid or conjunctiva. At the secondary stage, it may cause uveitis. Optic atrophy occurs as a complication of tertiary syphilis. In congenital syphilis, bilateral interstitial keratitis and chorioretinal scars may develop.

Tuberculosis

Many inflammatory ocular conditions, including scleritis and uveitis, are said to be associated with a focal tuberculous infection. However, it is unlikely that tuberculosis is a significant causative agent in these and other ocular diseases of unknown etiology.

OTHER CONDITIONS

Rheumatoid arthritis

Rheumatoid arthritis can affect the eyes in several ways. It may cause persistent irritation and congestion on account of dry eyes. Episcleritis is a common cause of localised redness of the eyes in rheumatoid patients. Scleritis may be localised, nodular or diffuse. When severe, there is necrosis of the sclera known as scleromalacia. Rheumatoid arthritis can also be complicated by long-term therapy with Chloroquine or steroids. Chloroquine can cause maculopathy and corneal deposits. Cataract may develop with long-term systemic steroid therapy.

Muco-cutaneous diseases

Acne rosacea may cause chronic conjunctivitis or blepharitis and more importantly, severe superficial keratitis with corneal vascularisation. It is usually bilateral with a tongue-like opacity of the cornea and, if it affects the pupillary region, severe visual loss will result. Acne rosacea is common among Caucasians in Europe. Treatment is with steroid eyedrops.

Stevens-Johnson's syndrome is an acute inflammation of the skin and mucous membrane. The eruptions are sometimes caused by a drug. The most common ocular manifestation is severe conjunctivitis which may result in corneal scarring with dry eyes and corneal opacity. Treatment with artificial tears, contact lenses and plastic surgical procedures may help.

Ear, nose and throat conditions

Infection of the paranasal sinuses may lead to orbital cellulitis. Unilateral proptosis sometimes develops from a mucocele of the sinus or from infiltration of the orbit by nasopharyngeal carcinoma, a common condition in the Chinese.

Diabetic Retinopathy — Background

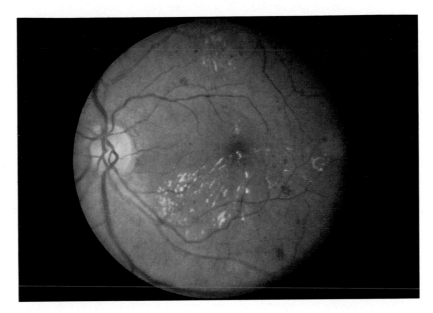

Fig. 6.1
Background diabetic retinopathy showing scattered exudates and haemorrhages near fovea. Normal vision (6/6). Laser photocoagulation indicated.

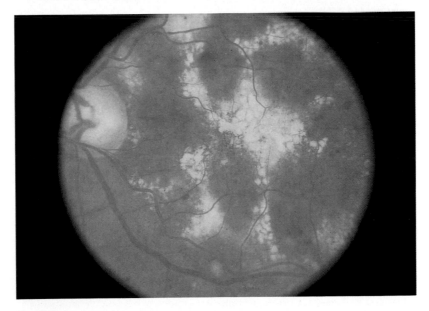

Fig. 6.2
Background diabetic retinopathy with severe maculopathy. Hard exudates at macula. Vision 6/60. Central vision permanently lost.

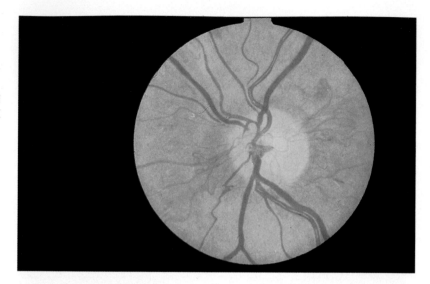

Fig. 6.3
Proliferative diabetic retinopathy with disc neovascularisation. Vision 6/6. Laser photocoagulation required.

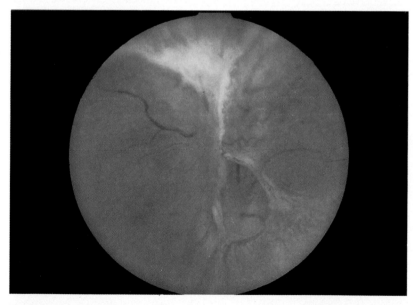

Fig. 6.4
Advanced proliferative diabetic retinopathy with traction retinal detachment resulting from preretinal scar tissue. Vision: hand movement. Too late for treatment.

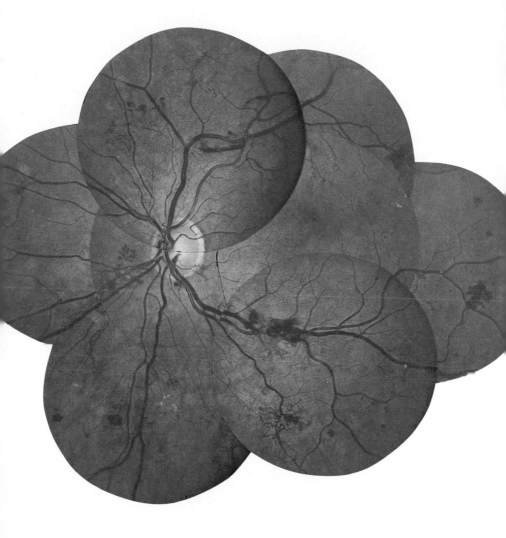

Fig. 6.5
Proliferative diabetic retinopathy with abnormal vessels at optic disc and retina
with early vitreous haemorrhage. Eye in danger of being blind and requires laser
photocoagulation.

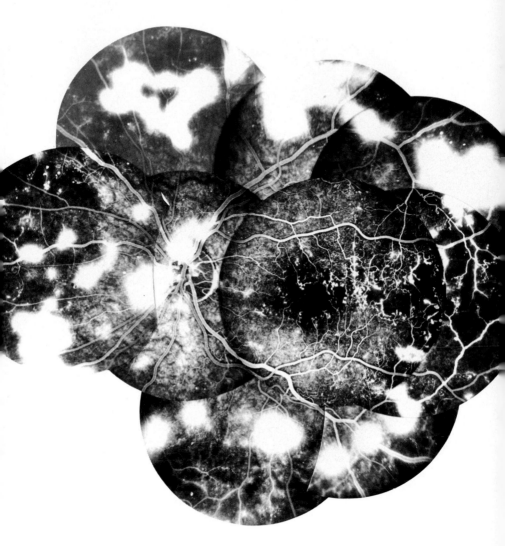

Fig. 6.6
Fundal fluorescein angiography showed extensive dye leaks at optic disc and retinal periphery. Abnormal capillaries and capillary fall-out. This emphasises importance of angiography in evaluation of retina as severity of retinopathy sometimes not obvious with ophthalmoscopy.

Photocoagulation

Photocoagulation combined with good metabolic control prevents more than 50% blindness resulting from diabetic retinopathy.

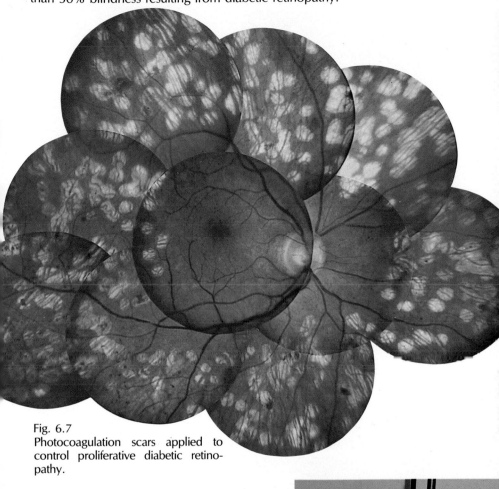

Fig. 6.7
Photocoagulation scars applied to control proliferative diabetic retinopathy.

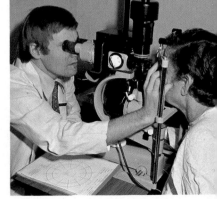

Fig. 6.8
Argon laser photocoagulator.

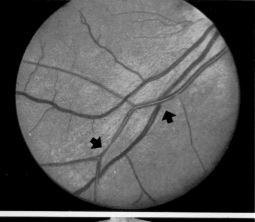

Fig. 6.9
Grade II hypertensive retinopathy with focal narrowing of artery and arteriovenous nipping.

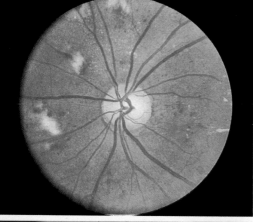

Fig. 6.10
Grade III hypertensive retinopathy with soft exudates, oedema and haemorrhages.

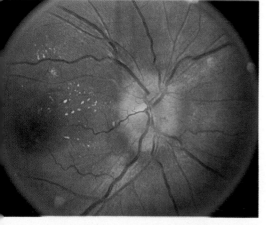

Fig. 6.11
Grade IV hypertensive retinopathy with papilloedema (malignant hypertension).

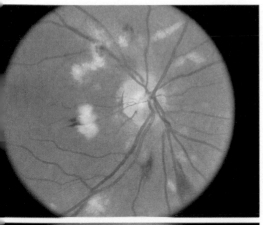

Fig. 6.12
Non-specific retinal haemorrhages with soft exudates seen in severe anaemia.

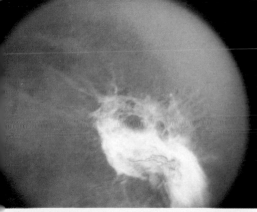

Fig. 6.13
Fibrous proliferations at retinal periphery seen in sickle-cell retinopathy.

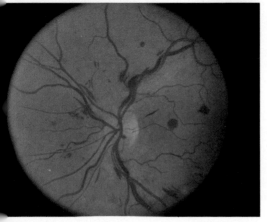

Fig. 6.14
Engorged and tortuous retinal veins seen in hyperviscosity retinopathy. Appearance similar to that of central retinal vein occlusion.

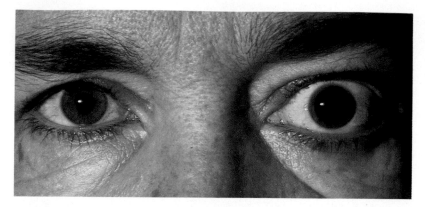

Fig. 6.15
Unilateral left exophthalmos
with lid retraction.

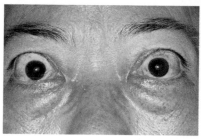

Fig. 6.16
Bilateral exophthalmos with
marked lid retraction.

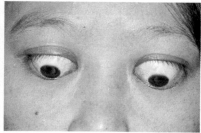

Fig. 6.17
Bilateral lid lag.

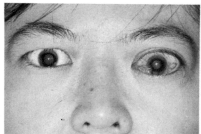

Fig. 6.18
Left exposure keratitis caused
by exophthalmos, lid retraction
and lagophthalmos (inability to
close eyelid).

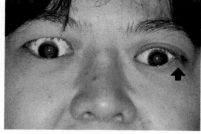

Fig. 6.19
Left lateral tarsorrhaphy to pro-
tect cornea. Same patient as in
Fig. 6.18.

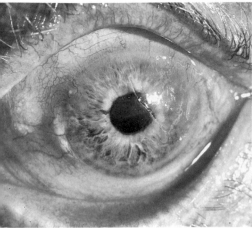

Fig. 6.20
Dry eye with loss of corneal lustre.

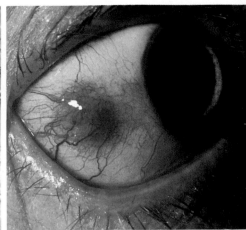

Fig. 6.21
Nodular scleritis.

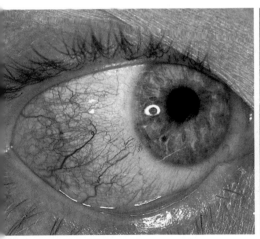

Fig. 6.22
Diffuse scleritis.

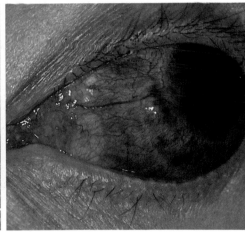

Fig. 6.23
Extensive scleromalacia with brown uveal tissue seen beneath thin sclera.

7

NEURO-OPHTHALMOLOGY

INTRODUCTION

The visual pathway or the third, fourth, fifth and sixth cranial nerves are frequently affected by diseases of the central nervous system. Because the clinical features are often sensitive indicators of neurological diseases, a special field of ophthalmology has developed — neuro-ophthalmology.

An important problem is to determine whether the optic disc swelling is due to papilloedema, papillitis or ischaemic optic neuropathy. Optic atrophy is a common clinical manifestation which requires diagnosis and a full neurological evaluation. A chiasmal lesion causes a bitemporal hemianopic field defect whereas a post-chiasmal lesion causes a homonymous field loss.

OPTIC DISC SWELLING

The ophthalmoscopic picture of optic disc swelling shows blurring of the disc margin and swelling of the optic nerve head, with filling in of the central physiological cup. The veins are dilated and venous pulsations are absent. There are often small superficial haemorrhages confined to the immediate disc area, and oedema of the surrounding retina. In early disc swelling, fundal fluorescein angiography may help to determine its presence.

Papilloedema or papillitis

The ophthalmoscopic appearance of disc oedema in papilloedema and papillitis is the same. Papilloedema is differentiated from papillitis by the presence of other clinical features.

Papilloedema is a passive swelling of the optic disc commonly caused by raised intracranial pressure. The condition is usually bilateral. Vision is normal unless the macula is affected by oedema or exudates. Rarely is the vision diminished because of optic atrophy in severe unrelieved papilloedema. The visual fields and colour vision are also normal although the blind spot is sometimes enlarged. The pupillary reflex to light is normal.

Papillitis is an inflammation of the optic nerve, frequently of uncertain aetiology. Disseminated sclerosis is an important cause. The condition is usually unilateral. Because the optic nerve is inflamed, there is usually marked visual loss. A central scotoma is present and the eye may have defective colour vision, especially to red. The pupil is dilated, with sluggish or no reaction to direct light.

	PAPILLOEDEMA	PAPILLITIS
Visual Acuity	Normal (usually)	Reduced
Pupil	Normal	Dilated and shows poor response to direct light
Visual Field	Normal (increased blind spot)	Central scotoma or field defect
Colour Vision	Normal	Defective
	Usually bilateral	Usually unilateral

Differential diagnosis of papilloedema and papillitis.

Ischaemic optic neuropathy

Ischaemia to the optic nerve head from arteriolar sclerosis and temporal arteritis also causes sudden visual loss with a swollen optic disc in the elderly population. It is important to exclude temporal arteritis by blood erythrocyte sedimentation rate (ESR). Systemic steroids will protect the unaffected eye. The prognosis for the affected eye is usually poor and optic atrophy usually follows.

Pseudo-papilloedema

Pseudo-papilloedema is a variation in the appearance of the optic disc which is sometimes mistaken for true disc oedema. It should be clearly differentiated from the latter in order to avoid unnecessary investigations and anxiety to the patient.

One common cause of pseudo-papilloedema is hypermetropia where the disc margin is blurred. Other common causes include drusen (yellowish-white deposits at the optic disc) and opaque myelinated nerve fibres. Fundal fluorescein angiography can help to distinguish pseudo-papilloedema from true disc oedema.

RETROBULBAR NEURITIS

Retrobulbar neuritis is an inflammation of the optic nerve with similar symptoms and signs as papillitis except that the optic disc oedema is absent. The clinical features include pain on movement of the eyes, sudden blurred vision, defective colour vision and a central scotoma. The cause is usually unknown but some patients have underlying disseminated sclerosis. There is no specific treatment. Steroids may be used to speed up recovery of the central vision.

OPTIC ATROPHY

Because the colour of the optic disc varies in normal individuals, a pale optic disc does not necessarily signify the presence of optic atrophy. Optic atrophy is confirmed where a pale optic disc is associated with defective visual acuity and visual field.

There are numerous causes of optic atrophy and they include optic neuritis, meningitis, encephalitis, central retinal artery occlusion, chronic ischaemia of the optic nerve, compression of the optic nerve or chiasma, trauma, chronic glaucoma, retinitis pigmentosa, congenital and familial disorders, and exogenous factors such as toxic processes, malnutrition, Vitamin B deficiency and syphilis. The cause is frequently undetermined.

Neurological investigations must be carried out to exclude compression of the optic nerve by intracranial tumours and other treatable causes.

CHIASMAL LESION

A chiasmal lesion causes a characteristic bitemporal hemianopic field defect. A chromophobe adenoma is the most common cause. The presence of optic atrophy and poor visual acuity usually indicates that the condition is already at a very advanced stage. Diagnosis is made by finding the characteristic field defect and confirmed by radiology of the skull. It should be differentiated from other causes of a chiasmal lesion such as a suprasellar cyst (craniopharyngioma) or meningioma.

Post-chiasmal lesion

A post-chiasmal lesion causes a homonymous hemianopic field defect. It is usually due to either a cerebro-vascular occlusion or a tumour. The optic tract, the optic radiation or the visual cortex may be affected. If the lesion is further back at the occipital lobe, the homonymous hemianopia tends to be congruous (similar). If the lesion occurs further forward and affects the optic tract, the homonymous hemianopia will tend to be incongruous (dissimilar). At the optic radiation, a homonymous quadrantic field defect may occur because the visual pathway is spread out over a relatively large area.

Computerized tomography and nuclear magnetic resonance scans

CT scan and now NMR are commonly used in neuro-ophthalmic investigations. They permit accurate localisation of pathology affecting the visual pathway. These investigations are also particularly valuable in evaluating the extent of intracranial lesions.

PUPILS

The pupils may be abnormal in size or shape or in their reaction to light and accommodation.

Large pupil

A large pupil may be caused by mydriatic eyedrops, optic neuritis, optic atrophy and oculomotor nerve paralysis. It may also be caused by blunt injury to the eye which has damaged the pupillary sphincter (traumatic mydriasis), or by advanced disease of the retina. Less commonly, it is due to Adie's tonic pupil.

Small pupil

A small pupil can be caused by miotic eyedrops such as Pilocarpine. Other causes include iritis, Horner's syndrome (sympathetic paralysis), Argyll Robertson pupil due to syphilis and morphine.

Irregular pupil

A pupil which is irregular may be due to a congenital iris defect, posterior synechiae from iritis, Argyll Robertson pupil, or surgery.

Reaction to light

A pupil which is not reactive to direct light but which is reactive to consensual light suggests that the eye is severely damaged or blind from disease of the retina or the optic nerve (Marcus Gunn pupil). A pupil which is not reactive to either direct or consensual light indicates local disease or injury to the sphincter of the iris, or damage to the third cranial nerve, the nerve supply of the pupillary sphincter. Sometimes it is due to the use of a mydriatic.

In the Argyll Robertson pupil there is no reaction to light but the pupils react to accommodation.

EXTRAOCULAR MUSCLES

Paralytic squints

In severe paralysis of the extraocular muscles, the diagnosis is usually obvious. Lesions of the third nerve lead to ptosis and a relatively immobile eyeball which deviates downwards and outwards. This deviation is due to the paralysis of all the extraocular muscles except for the lateral rectus and the superior oblique. The pupil is dilated.

In lesions of the sixth nerve, there will be a convergent squint. In lesions of the fourth nerve, the superior oblique muscle is paralysed. The eye is elevated when it is in an adducted position because of the overaction of the inferior oblique muscle. The patient often has a compensatory head posture to avoid double vision.

Numerous conditions may result in paralysis of the extraocular muscles. The cause is often difficult to determine and special investigation may be required. Trauma, diabetes, arteriosclerosis, intracranial aneurysms and tumours are the most common causes.

In slight paralysis the ocular movements are apparently normal. The patient complains of double vision and the diagnosis can be difficult. The following simple questions may help to confirm the presence of muscle paralysis.

- Is double vision present when both eyes are open? Is double vision present when one eye is closed? Extraocular muscle paralysis causes binocular double vision. If double vision is present when one eye is occluded, it is not due to paralysis of the extraocular muscles.

- Does the separation of images occur side by side or one above the other? In sixth nerve paralysis the separation is side by side while in third or fourth nerve paralysis the separation is one above the other.

- In which direction of gaze does the maximum separation occur? Maximum separation of images occurs in the direction of action of the affected muscle. For example, there will be maximum separation of images when the patient looks to the left if the left lateral rectus muscle is affected.

- In which eye is the image fainter? The fainter image is seen by the eye with the paralysed muscle. If there is left lateral rectus muscle paralysis, there will be a horizontal separation of images and the fainter image is seen with the left eye.

The cover test for diagnosis of strabismus and special optical tests are required to investigate patients with diplopia and to chart their progress.

Myasthenia gravis

Myasthenia gravis causes weakness of the skeletal muscles, especially in young adults. The extraocular muscles are frequently affected. Thus, the patient may present with intermittent and varying double vision and ptosis which is usually bilateral. The symptoms are classically more pronounced in the evening. They can be precipitated clinically by asking the patient to keep a sustained upward gaze for a minute or two.

Diagnosis can be confirmed by demonstrating a reversal of symptoms with intravenous tensilon.

NYSTAGMUS

Nystagmus is an involuntary, oscillatory movement of the eyes.

Jerk nystagmus has a slow and fast component and is usually maximum in a particular position of gaze. It is caused by neurological conditions which affect either the cerebellum, the vestibular system or their connections. Patients with jerk nystagmus require a full neurological evaluation.

Ocular (pendular) nystagmus has no slow or fast component. It is caused by poor vision and the patient's inability to fix his gaze. As a result the eye develops a pendular movement.

Both jerk and pendular nystagmus are often congenital.

Migraine

Migraine is a common cause of headaches. Often there is visual disturbance prior to the onset of the unilateral headache. This presents as sparkling or flashing lights followed by a positive field defect. The symptoms are all unilateral. The headache is frequently associated with nausea and vomiting. The symptoms are usually relieved by resting quietly in a darkened room combined with the administration of vaso-dilators. There is frequently a family history of migraine. Occasionally migraine-like attacks are due to pathological lesions such as intracranial aneurysms and tumours. Severe, atypical persistent migraine or migraine of late onset require neurological investigation.

Disc Oedema

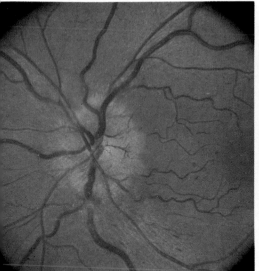

Fig. 7.1
Papillitis due to inflammation.

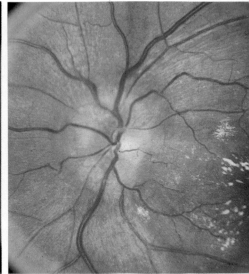

Fig. 7.2
Papilloedema due to malignant hypertension.

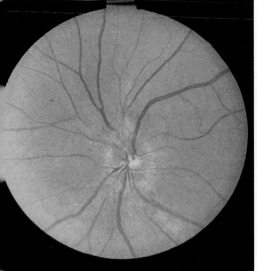

Fig. 7.3
Blurred disc margin suggesting possible disc oedema.

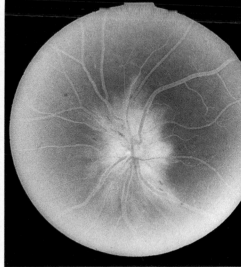

Fig. 7.4
Fundal fluorescein angiography confirms disc oedema. (Same eye as in Fig. 7.3)

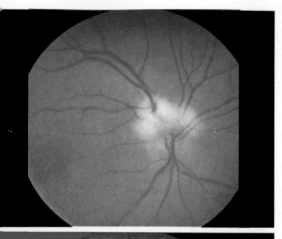

Fig. 7.5
Opaque nerve fibres.

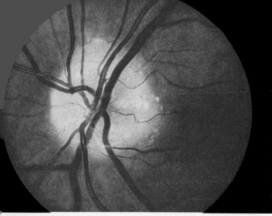

Fig. 7.6
Disc drusen.

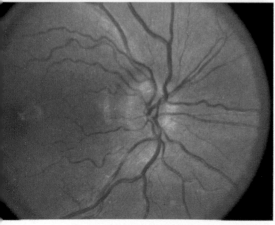

Fig. 7.7
Hypermetropia with small optic disc and blurred margins.

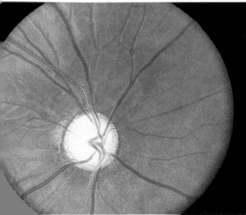

Fig. 7.8
Optic atrophy of undetermined aetiology.

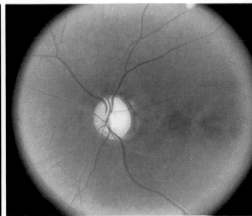

Fig. 7.9
Optic atrophy following central retinal
artery occlusion (same eye as in Fig.
5.1 a year later).

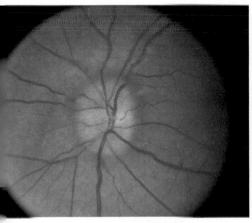

Fig. 7.10
Optic atrophy following papillitis, with
blurred margin.

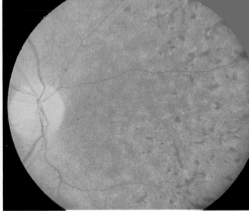

Fig. 7.11
Optic atrophy in retinitis pigmentosa,
with yellow-white optic disc and
attenuated retinal vessels.

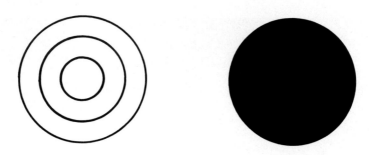

Fig. 7.12
Right optic atrophy with complete field loss.

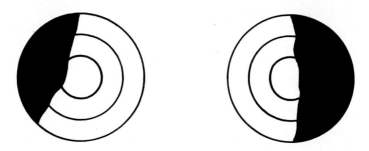

Fig. 7.13
Bitemporal field defect indicating lesion at chiasma.

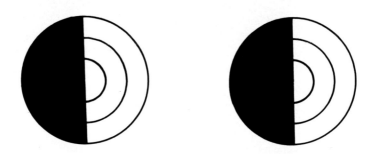

Fig. 7.14
Homonymous (left) field defect indicating post-chiasmal lesion.

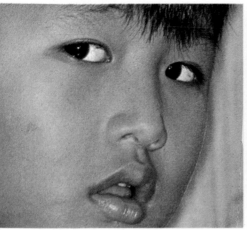

Fig. 7.15
Right superior oblique muscle paralysis leading to head tilt to avoid double vision.

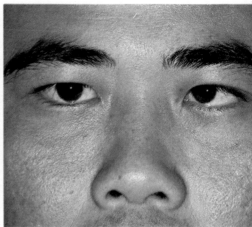

Fig. 7.16
Left lateral rectus paralysis causing convergent squint.

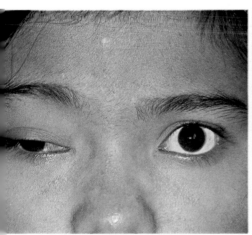

Fig. 7.17
Right third nerve paralysis causing ptosis and divergent squint.

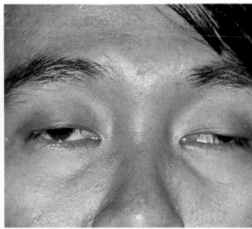

Fig. 7.18
Bilateral ptosis and divergent squint in myasthenia gravis.

Complete Third Nerve Paralysis

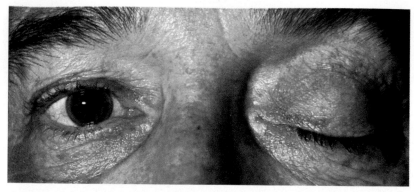

Fig. 7.19
Complete left ptosis (looking straight ahead).

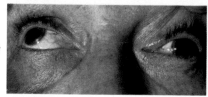

Fig. 7.20
Left inferior oblique paralysis (looking up and right).

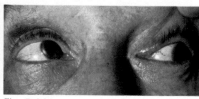

Fig. 7.21
Left superior rectus paralysis (looking up and left).

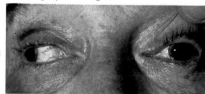

Fig. 7.22
Left medial rectus paralysis (looking right).

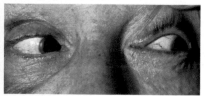

Fig. 7.23
Normal left lateral rectus (looking left).

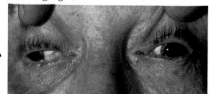

Fig. 7.24
Left superior oblique action is limited (because of inability to adduct: looking down and right).

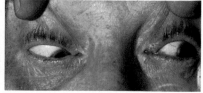

Fig. 7.25
Left inferior rectus paralysis (looking down and left).

Note: Third cranial nerve supplies levator palpebrae superioris besides medial, superior and inferior rectus and inferior oblique muscles.

8

EYE DISEASES IN CHILDREN

INTRODUCTION

A rare but important ocular condition in children is retino-blastoma, a malignant tumour which usually presents as a "white pupil". Early diagnosis may save the life of the child.

Squint is common in children, especially in Caucasians, and should be evaluated and treated early to prevent loss of vision from amblyopia (lazy eye).

Other common conditions include conjunctivitis, blocked nasolacrimal duct and congenital cataract.

WHITE PUPIL (DIFFERENTIAL DIAGNOSIS)

- Retinoblastoma
- Retinopathy of prematurity (retrolental fibroplasia). In this condition, there is a history of prematurity and the use of oxygen.
- Dense congenital cataract. This is easily recognised.
- Persistent primary hyperplastic vitreous. The eye is abnormally small.
- Coats' disease. There is massive exudates from abnormal retinal vessels.
- Endophthalmitis (inflammation of the whole eye due to infections).
- Organised vitreous haemorrhage.

Retinoblastoma

Retinoblastoma is an important cause of the white pupil (cat's eye reflex) in children. Usually, the condition is detected when an abnormal whiteness appears in the child's pupil. This is most obvious in dim light when the pupil is partially dilated. In most cases, the presence of the white reflex indicates that the condition is at an advanced stage.

As retinoblastoma is highly malignant and can spread rapidly, it must be differentiated from other causes of a white pupil.

The differential diagnosis can be difficult even for an experienced ophthalmologist. A child with a white pupil should be urgently referred to an ophthalmologist to establish the cause. Examination under general anaesthesia with full dilatation of the pupils is required to determine the diagnosis and exclude retinoblastoma.

Management

An eye with a retinoblastoma usually requires removal as soon as possible. As retinoblastoma frequently affects the fellow eye, this should also be examined under anaesthesia with full dilatation of the pupil. These examinations have to be repeated at regular intervals. If early retinoblastoma is found, it can be treated with a combination of radio-therapy, photocoagulation and cryoapplication.

Retinopathy of prematurity

All premature babies, especially those who require oxygen, should have their fundus examined by an ophthalmologist for early signs of retinopathy. Oxygen causes constriction and obliteration of premature blood vessels in the peripheral retina. This leads to new vessel proliferation exudation, scarring and retinal detachment. Treatment by photocoagulation, cryotherapy or even vitreous surgery may be indicated.

SQUINTS IN CHILDREN

Squint is a deviation of an eye, so that its visual axis is no longer parallel with that of its fellow eye. In a convergent squint, one of the eyes is turned inwards, while in a divergent squint one of the eyes is turned outwards. Deviation of the eyes may also be vertical, with one eye higher than the other. This is known as a vertical squint.

Squints may be due to paralysis of a muscle (paralytic squint) or there may be no obvious evidence of paralysis (non-paralytic or concomitant squint). In a paralytic squint the degree of deviation of the eyes is not the same in all fields of gaze. In a non-paralytic or concomitant squint the degree of deviation is the same in all directions of gaze.

Paralytic squints

The ocular manifestations of paralytic squints in children are generally similar to those in adults, except that the child does not complain of double vision. To avoid double vision, the child suppresses the use of one eye, leading to amblyopia. Sometimes, the child adopts a compensatory head tilt to avoid double vision.

Non-paralytic squints

Non-paralytic squints may be convergent or divergent. Sometimes, one of the eyes is higher, in which case there is a vertical element.

A convergent squint is often associated with hypermetropia (long sight). Correction of the hypermetropia with glasses can reduce the squint. This type of squint is known as accommodative convergent squint. It is common in Caucasian children but not in other races. A divergent squint in a child usually develops after the age of three years and is often associated with myopia.

Frequently, a non-paralytic squint is precipitated by illnesses such as measles or chicken pox. An important consideration in young children is that the squint may occasionally be due to poor vision or secondary to ocular disease, of which retinoblastoma is the most important.

Effects of squint on children

There are three effects of squint on children:
- Amblyopia (lazy eye).
- Failure to develop binocular single vision.
- Cosmetic blemish. This can lead to emotional and socio-economic problems.

Management

The child should be referred to an ophthalmologist as soon as a squint is suspected for exclusion of ocular pathology, especially retinoblastoma, and to commence treatment for amblyopia.

Refraction with Atropine or other cycloplegics should be carried out and, where necessary, appropriate glasses prescribed. Glasses for children with accommodative convergent squint may be adequate to correct the squint and these glasses should be used constantly.

Early diagnosis and treatment may prevent the development of amblyopia or increase the chances of reversing it. Treatment includes patching of the good eye until maximum improvement of the amblyopic eye is obtained. This is usually supervised by an orthoptist. Patching can be tedious, and needs the co-operation of the child and its parents.

Surgery may be necessary. In a convergent squint, surgery is directed at weakening the medial rectus muscle and strengthening the lateral rectus muscle. The opposite procedure is done in a divergent squint.

In squints which have a vertical element, surgery becomes more complicated as it involves surgery on one of the vertically acting muscles, that is, the superior or inferior rectus, or one of the oblique muscles. Although it is usual for the eyes to be straightened at one operation, it may occasionally require more than one operation.

It is important to explain to the parents that even after surgery to straighten the eyes, patching of the good eye and continued supervision are required.

Amblyopia

Amblyopia is an important condition in children and is present in up to 5% of some populations. In a squint, whether paralytic or non-paralytic, the child suppresses the use of one eye in order to avoid double vision. Persistent suppression of the eye causes amblyopia, (sometimes referred to as a lazy eye).

It is important to treat a child with squint as early as possible since amblyopia can frequently be prevented or reversed by patching the good eye to stimulate the squinting eye to function.

Refractive amblyopia is due to anisometropia (difference of refraction in each eye), bilateral high astigmatism or hypermetropia (long-sight). Amblyopia can also be caused by ptosis, corneal scar, cataract or congenital nystagmus.

Pseudo-squint

Pseudo-squint is usually due to marked medial epicanthal eyelid folds which give the appearance of a convergent squint. Diagnosis is confirmed by observing the corneal reflex and the cover test. As the child grows older, the skin folds tend to become less marked. No treatment, only reassurance, is required.

INFECTIOUS CONJUNCTIVITIS

Conjunctivitis occurring in the first twenty-eight days after birth is referred to as ophthalmia neonatorum. In the past, the infection was usually due to gonorrhoea. In recent years, better antenatal care in most countries has made gonorrhoea less common. Other causative organisms include staphylococcus, streptococcus, haemophilus, pneumococcus, coliform organisms, herpes simplex virus and chlamydia, (TRIC organism found in the genital tract of females).

In gonococcal infection, there is acute purulent conjunctivitis which can perforate the cornea and lead to blindness.

If the conjunctivitis is severe, urgent treatment with systemic and local therapy is required. The child may have to be hospitalised with barrier nursing to prevent the spread of the infection. However, many milder cases of conjunctivitis can be treated as outpatients with hourly applications of antibiotic eyedrops until the infection clears. It is important to clean the discharge regularly with sterile (boiled) cotton wool, soaked in saline or water.

LACRIMAL SYSTEM (TEARING)

Blockage of the lacrimal drainage system in a child usually occurs at the nasolacrimal duct. Within the first few weeks of life one eye is noticed to water and to be stickier than the other. Pressure with the finger on the lacrimal sac often produces a reflux of mucopurulent material. This is due to late canalisation of the lacrimal drainage system which first develops as a solid cord of epithelial cells and normally canalises at about the time of birth. Occasionally, it is not a developmental abnormality but is due to blockage of the nasolacrimal duct by debris.

Treatment is conservative, with application of astringent eyedrops (Zinc sulphate 1/4%) and daily massage of the lacrimal sac with the pulp of the finger (with short nail) for the first six months. Antibiotics are used only where there is an infection. Most cases will clear. If the condition persists, or if the infection is recurrent or severe, the child should be referred to an ophthalmologist for syringing under general anaesthesia. If there is a blockage, it may be necessary to probe the nasolacrimal duct. Surgery to anastomosise the sac to the nasal mucosa (dacryocystorhinostomy) is rarely required in children.

CONGENITAL CATARACT

Congenital cataract with minimal lens change which does not interfere with vision usually requires no surgery. When it is bilateral and dense, surgery should be performed in the first six months. Dense congenital cataracts should therefore be referred for an ophthalmic opinion as soon as possible. Where the cataract is not dense and where there is a fair view of the fundus, the decision for surgery can be difficult. It is advisable to wait until the child is older, when visual acuity can be more accurately determined.

If the cataract is unilateral, removal is not indicated except for cosmetic reasons, because the opacity appears as an unsightly white reflex at the pupil. Therefore despite surgery an eye with a unilateral cataract presenting in early childhood usually remains amblyopic.

Surgery involves aspiration of the lens after opening the anterior capsule under the operating microscope. This is possible because the nucleus of the child's lens is soft.

CONGENITAL GLAUCOMA

Congenital glaucoma is rare. In infants, raised intraocular pressure causes the cornea to increase in diameter from 11 mm to over 13 mm. Because of the increase in size, this condition is also known as buphthalmos (ox eye). It causes tears in the Descemet's membrane, leading to corneal oedema, irritation and watering of the eye combined with photophobia. If left unrelieved, the raised intraocular pressure with damage the optic nerve, resulting in glaucomatous cupping and optic atrophy.

Referral to an ophthalmologist of an infant with photophobia and tearing or a large and opaque cornea enables early diagnosis and treatment, and may prevent blindness. Surgery and life-long follow-up is necessary.

PHAKOMATOSES

This is a group of congenital or hereditary abnormalities which affect the skin, the nervous system and also the eye in varying degrees.

Neurofibromatosis (von Recklinghausen's disease) is characterised by pigmented patches of the skin (cafe-au-lait spots) and subcutaneous tumours of varying sizes. The brain stem or cerebellum may be affected by the tumours. The ocular manifestations include neurofibromas in the eyelids, orbit, retina and optic nerve gliomas.

Tuberous sclerosis (Bourneville's disease) is a disease in which gliomas of the brain are associated with sebaceous adenoma of the face. These are distributed across the nose and face in a typical butterfly pattern. Occasionally, the retina or optic disc has a yellowish raised nodule which looks like a mulberry.

Sturge-Weber syndrome is a capillary haemangioma or "portwine stain" affecting the distribution of the fifth nerve on the face. Capillary haemangioma may also affect the cerebral cortex. Sometimes, the eye on the side of the lesion, develops congenital glaucoma which can be difficult to treat. Choroidal angioma may also be present.

Von Hippel-Lindau disease is a condition with an elevated haemangioma at the retinal periphery associated with large feeding retinal vessels. Many have associated cerebellar or brain stem haemangioma. The haemangioma often causes exudates and haemorrhages in the retina and vitreous and can lead to retinal detachment. The retinal lesions should be treated with photocoagulation, diathermy or cryoapplication.

DEVELOPMENTAL ABNORMALITIES

There are a large number of developmental abnormalities which occur in mild or severe forms. The mechanism is not fully known. Some are associated with antenatal infections, teratogenic drugs and chromosomal abnormalities or hereditary defective genes.

The abnormalities may affect the whole skull and face, giving rise to a number of syndromes such as craniofacial dysostosis, mandibulo-facial dysostosis and meningo-encephalocele.

The whole eye may be affected in anophthalmos (absence of one eye, congenital cyst and microphthalmos — small eye). Coloboma of the iris or choroid is due to the absence of a part of the eye as a result of incomplete closure of the choroidal fissure.

Common abnormalities which affect the lids include congenital ptosis, coloboma of the lid and obstruction of the lacrimal apparatus.

The lens may be abnormal in shape or dislocated as in Marfan's syndrome and homocystinuria. Persistent hyaloid (embryonic vitreous) artery and hyperplastic primary vitreous which presents itself as a white pupil may also occur.

A number of abnormalities may occur at the optic disc. These include optic pits and hypoplasia of the optic nerve, which is an occasional cause of poor vision in childhood.

ANTENATAL INFECTIONS

Antenatal infection can lead to congenital syphilis, rubella or toxoplasmosis. The common manifestations of rubella are congenital cataract and nystagmus. Both syphilis and rubella can cause pigmentary changes of the retina. Congenital toxoplasmosis causes a typical localised pigmented chorioretinal scar at the macula.

Retinoblastoma

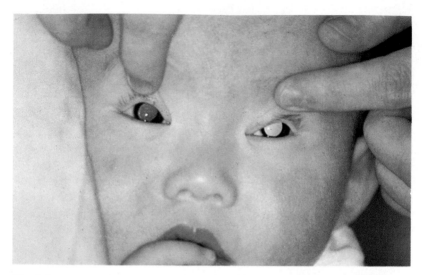

Fig. 8.1
Retinoblastoma in both eyes (note normal anterior segment).

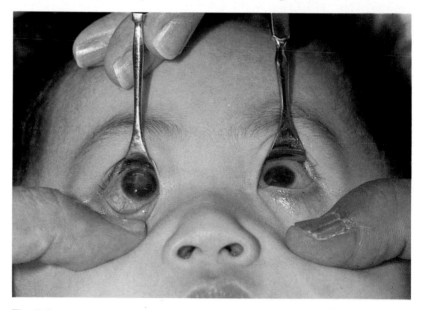

Fig. 8.2
Retrolental fibroplasia (note microcornea of left eye).

Convergent Squint

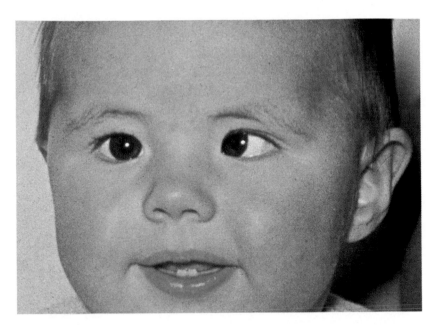

Fig. 8.3
Left congenital convergent squint.

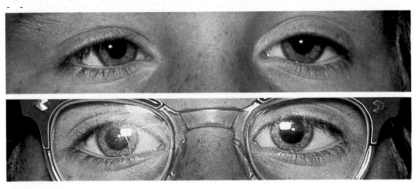

Fig. 8.4
Right convergent squint resulting from retinoblastoma (note white pupil).

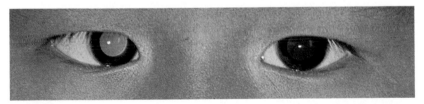

Fig. 8.5a & Fig. 8.5b
Right accommodative convergent squint straightened with hypermetropic glasses.

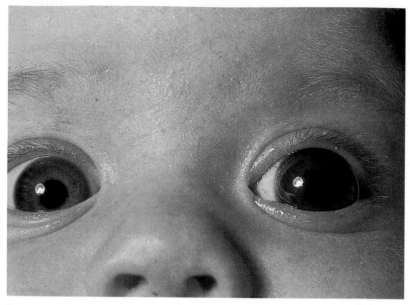

Fig. 8.6
Congenital glaucoma with enlarged corneal diameter, (buphthalmos or "ox eye")
especially left.

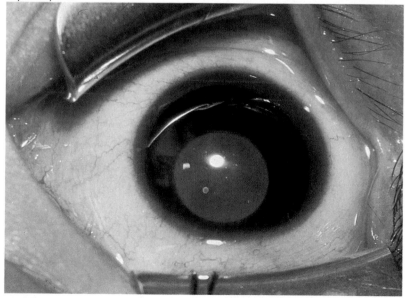

Fig. 8.7
Congenital cataract affecting nucleus of lens.

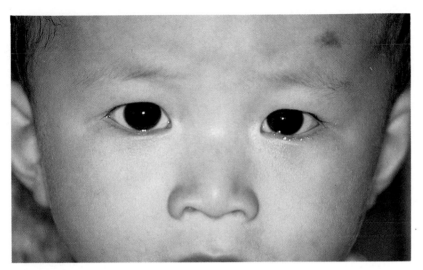

Fig. 8.8
Watering due to congenital blocked nasolacrimal duct.

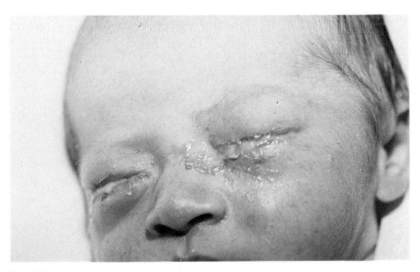

Fig. 8.9
Ophthalmia neonatorum.

(Courtesy of Dr Cheah Way Mun, Singapore.)

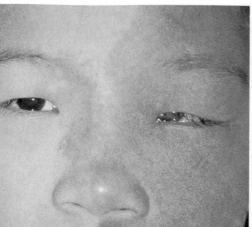

Fig. 8.10
Capillary haemangioma of left side of face with unilateral glaucoma in Sturge-Weber syndrome.

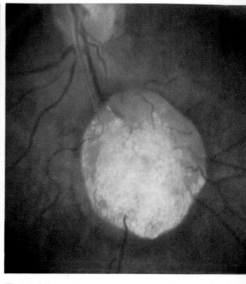

Fig. 8.11
Globular retinal tumour in tuberous sclerosis.

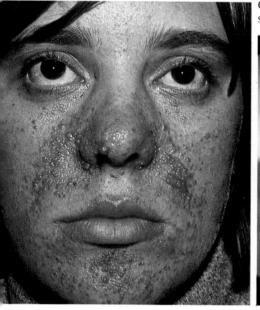

Fig. 8.13
Elevated globular haemangioma with large feeding retinal vessels in von Hippel-Lindau disease.

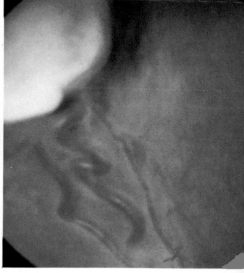

Fig. 8.12
Typical butterfly distribution of sebaceous adenoma.

Developmental Abnormality

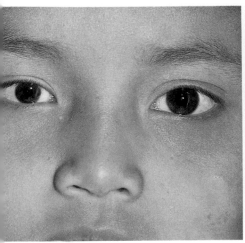

Fig. 8.14
Right microphthalmos.

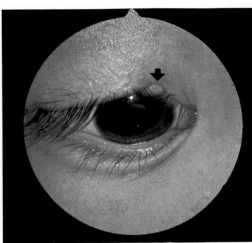

Fig. 8.15
Congenital coloboma of right upper lid.

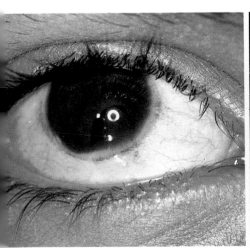

Fig. 8.16
Inferior nasal coloboma of iris.

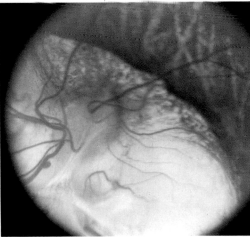

Fig. 8.17
Large choroidal coloboma involving optic disc and macula.

9

OCULAR INJURIES

INTRODUCTION

Ocular injuries are common. Some may be so trivial that only reassurance is required. On the other hand, some injuries are so severe that the eye is inevitably lost.

Ocular injuries may be due to any of the following:
- *Chemical injury*
- *Injury from "flying" particles*
- *Injury from sharp instruments*
- *Blunt injury*
- *Ocular injury associated with head injury*
- *Welding burns*

Visual acuity is extremely important in the assessment of ocular injuries for evaluation and for medico-legal reasons. The eye should be systematically examined. However, when a large penetrating wound of the cornea or sclera is suspected, it would be prudent not to examine the eye in detail, as a forceful examination may cause further ocular damage. Antibiotic eyedrops should be applied and the eye covered with a sterile eyepad. The patient should be referred immediately to an ophthalmologist.

PREVENTION

Many ocular injuries are preventable, and the physician may be in the best position to give advice.

Chemical injuries occur in laboratories and in chemical industries. Supervisors, teachers, students and workers should be warned that if any chemical gets into the eye, it should be immediately washed off with any available bland fluid or tap water. Protective eyeshields for those at risk should be used. Welding burns and injuries from "flying" particles in industries can be prevented by the use of goggles or special guards.

Intraocular foreign particle

When the velocity of the "flying" foreign particles is sufficiently great, the particle may penetrate the eyeball and cause loss of vision from:

- Direct damage, resulting in corneal opacity, hyphaema, cataract, vitreous haemorrhage or retinal trauma.
- Infection which may result in panophthalmitis.
- Any retained foreign particle, such as a piece of intraocular iron or copper particle which may disperse within the eyeball, causing irreversible damage.

On the other hand, glass particles are inert and may remain in the eye for years without causing any reaction.

A patient with an intraocular foreign body, apart from noticing that something has hit the eye, may have little to complain about. Because of this, it is important to carefully examine the patient under good lighting. X-rays must be taken if an intraocular foreign body is suspected. If there is any uncertainty, the patient should always be referred for an ophthalmic opinion.

Antibiotics should be given to prevent infection. If the intraocular foreign particle is made of iron or copper, it must be removed, as it will destroy the eyeball.

INJURY FROM SHARP INSTRUMENTS

Penetrating wound

A penetrating wound is usually due to a sharp or pointed instrument which has penetrated the eyeball. Loss of vision may be the result of direct damage to the cornea or to the lens, causing cataract. There may also be intraocular haemorrhage or retinal damage. The patient usually gives a history of a sharp or pointed instrument hitting the eye. It is important to obtain a precise history of the nature of the injury. The patient may complain of pain, watering eye and photophobia. The pupil is sometimes deformed due to a prolapsed iris.

Treatment is urgent. Antibiotic eyedrops are applied locally after the affected area has been cleaned. The eye should be covered with a sterile eyepad to immobilise the eyelids. It is unwise to try to examine the eye in detail, especially if there is a large penetrating wound, as the eye can be further damaged during examination. The patient should be referred immediately to an ophthalmologist as surgery is generally urgently required.

BLUNT INJURIES

Blunt injuries may damage the eye in many ways. Hyphaema is an important common injury. It is due to bleeding in the anterior chamber from a torn blood vessel in the iris. As the blood settles to the lowest part of the anterior chamber, a horizontal level of blood is seen. Often associated with this is a semi-dilated, immobile pupil known as "traumatic mydriasis" resulting from damage to the iris sphincter.

If neglected, further bleeding may occur leading to secondary glaucoma, and blood stained cornea. Because of this, hyphaema is an ocular emergency. The patient should be urgently referred for hospitalisation and bed-rest to prevent further bleeding.

If there is evidence of secondary glaucoma, surgery may be necessary to evacuate the blood clot from the anterior chamber.

Other complications which may develop from a blunt injury are cataract, dislocation of the lens, damage to the macula, vitreous haemorrhage and retinal detachment. Because so many structures may be damaged, patients with severe blunt injuries of the eye should be referred for ocular assessment as soon as possible.

Blowout fracture

A blunt injury sometimes does not injure the eyeball itself, but may instead fracture one of the thin walls of the orbit, usually the floor. This will cause the contents of the orbit to protrude into the maxillary antrum. The inferior rectus and inferior oblique muscles may be involved and result in double vision and limited elevation of the eye. Further evaluation is necessary and surgery is usually required.

OCULAR INJURY ASSOCIATED WITH HEAD INJURY

An ocular injury associated with a head injury is sometimes overlooked because the lid swelling makes it difficult to examine the eye and also attention is often diverted to other problems.

In patients, with severe head injuries, especially if there is bruising around the orbit, it is important to carry out a careful examination of the eyes and orbits.

Ocular injuries include damage to:
- Orbital wall — blowout fracture
- Optic nerve
- Extraocular muscles or their nerve supply
- Ocular structures

Welding burn (Arc burn)

Within eight hours following exposure to intense ultraviolet light, the worker and even those observing the job may complain of severe photophobia, blepharospasm, pain and watering of the eyes.

A drop of local anaesthetic can be used to facilitate examination to ensure that the symptoms are not due to some other injury. Treatment consists of relieving the symptoms of pain and photophobia with analgesics and patching of the eyes. Use of local anaesthetic drugs for pain relief should be avoided. This condition usually subsides in twenty-four hours.

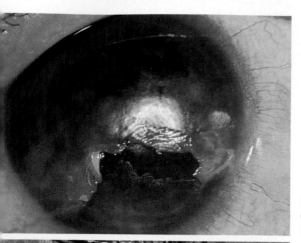

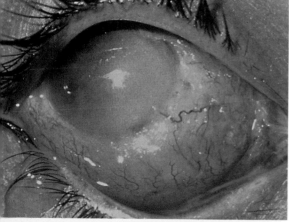

Fig. 9.1
Chemical burn typically affecting the cornea inferiorly.

Fig. 9.2
Corneal opacity following lime burn.

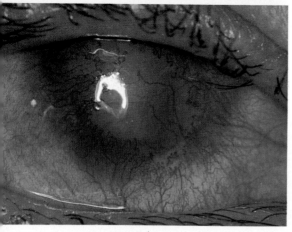

Fig. 9.3
Opaque vascularised cornea after severe chemical burn.

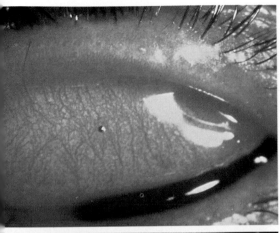

Fig. 9.4
Foreign particle on upper tarsal conjunctiva (everted upper lid).

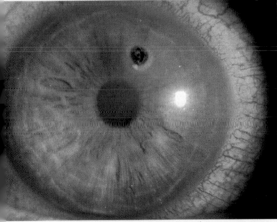

Fig. 9.5
Foreign particle on cornea.

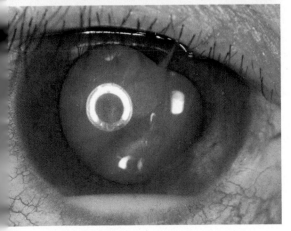

Fig. 9.6
Intraocular foreign body causing cataract and infection with hypopyon (pus in anterior chamber).

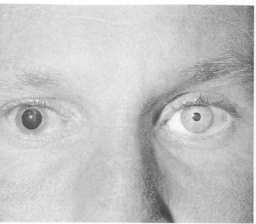

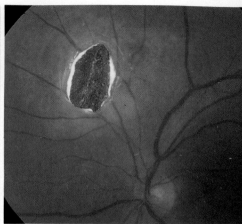

Fig. 9.7
Siderosis bulbi of right eye caused by retained iron particle in eye.

Fig. 9.8
Iron particle in vitreous.

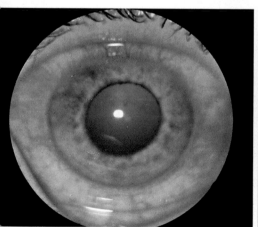

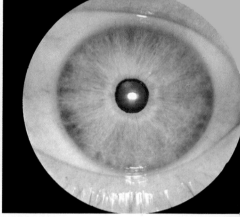

Fig. 9.9
Siderosis bulbi of right eye. Iris colour changed to brown (same patient as in Fig. 9.7).

Fig. 9.10
Left eye normal (same patient as in Fig. 9.7).

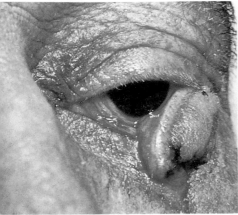

Fig. 9.11
Laceration of lower lid involving inferior canaliculus.

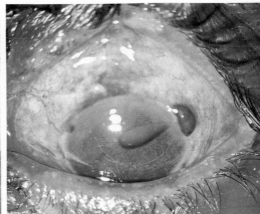

Fig. 9.12
Penetrating corneal laceration with prolapse of iris. Note distorted pupil.

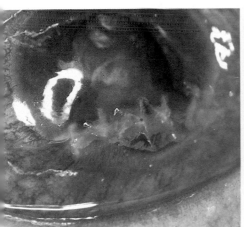

Fig. 9.13
Lacerated cornea with cataract.

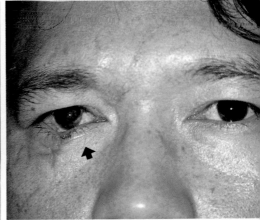

Fig. 9.14
Lacerated eyelids, cornea and sclera following motor-car accident.

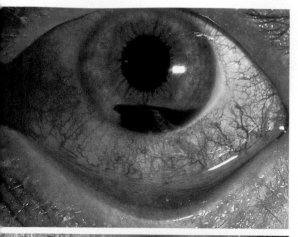

Fig. 9.15
Small hyphaema (blood in anterior chamber) — characteristic fluid level of blood.

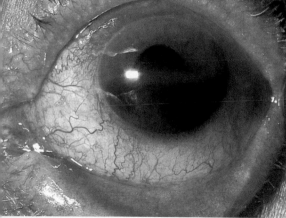

Fig. 9.16
Hyphaema filling more than half anterior chamber.

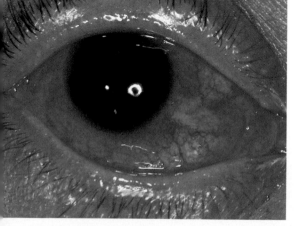

Fig. 9.17
Hyphaema filling entire anterior chamber complicated by secondary glaucoma.

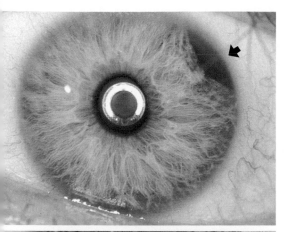

Fig. 9.18
Iridodialysis — iris torn at root.

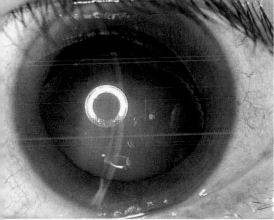

Fig. 9.19
Dislocated lens.

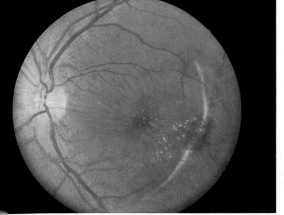

Fig. 9.20
Commotio retinae (traumatic oedema of macula) with typical curved choroidal tear, temporal to macula.

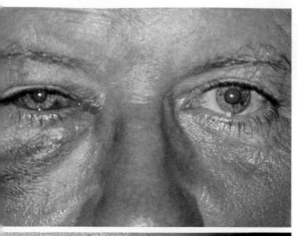

Fig. 9.21
Right lower-lid haematoma and oedema with subconjunctival haemorrhage.

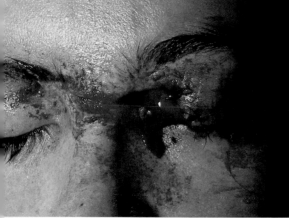

Fig. 9.22
Multiple lacerations of lids and face by glass fragments in motor-car accident (without seat belt). Cornea also lacerated.

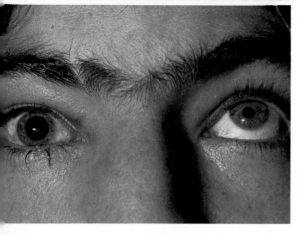

Fig. 9.23
Right blow-out fracture with limited elevation of right eye (right pupil dilated with mydriatics).

10

REFRACTIVE ERRORS

INTRODUCTION

A common cause of blurred vision is refractive error. This is a physiological condition where the refracting system of the eye fails to focus objects sharply on the retina. It is usually corrected with glasses. A useful rapid test to distinguish between refractive error and disease of the eye is the use of a pin-hole.

In modern societies, contact lenses are sometimes preferred to glasses mainly for cosmetic reasons. When contact lenses are used, it is important for the wearer to take the necessary precautions to prevent complications as serious ocular damage may occasionally develop.

REFRACTIVE ERROR

Myopia

Myopia (short sight) is an optical condition where distant objects are focused in front of the retina so that vision for distance is blurred but near vision is normal. Myopia is more common in the orientals. It is a common cause of blurred vision. Glasses are the usual way to correct this and they are usually prescribed by an ophthalmologist or an optometrist. Contact lenses are also a popular and efficient means of correcting myopia. Myopia is more common in the orientals. Recently, radial keratotomy has became a popular method to correct simple myopia in some countries. Its use is still controversial.

Common myopia is known as simple myopia, and is not associated with any degenerative changes at the retina. It is important to distinguish simple myopia from degenerative myopia. Simple myopia does not lead to visual loss. It is a physiological condition which can be fully corrected optically.

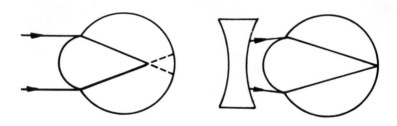

Fig. 10.1
Simple myopia corrected with a concave lens.

Hypermetropia

Hypermetropia (long sight) is a condition where a distant object is focused behind the retina. In the young, because of the strong accommodative power of the lens, hypermetropia is compensated. With age however, the power of accommodation decreases and the patient soon finds that he is unable to compensate. This begins with difficulty in focusing for near vision and later, for distance. Because of this, the patient requires the use of reading glasses earlier in life. With time, glasses are required for distant vision as well.

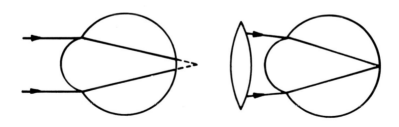

Fig. 10.2
Hypermetropia corrected with a convex lens.

Astigmatism

Astigmatism is a condition where the image cannot be focused sharply on a point because either the cornea or the lens is not spherical and has greater power in one meridian. Marked astigmatism causes poor vision for both distance and near. It is corrected with a cylindrical lens. A cylinder is shaped like a food can with no power in one axis and maximum power at right angles to that axis. Sometimes the astigmatism is irregular. This is caused by corneal scarring or by keratoconus (conical cornea). Irregular astigmatism is usually difficult to correct with glasses. Contact lenses frequently help.

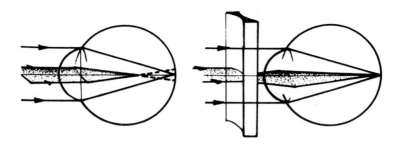

Fig. 10.3
Astigmatism corrected with a cylindrical lens.

Presbyopia

Presbyopia (old-age sight) is a condition of weak accommodation brought about by age. A young child has considerable ability to accommodate. This diminishes because of the progressive weakness in accommodation and near vision becomes progressively worse. Glasses for near vision are required even though the distant vision is perfect. For persons who require a correction for both distance and near in a single pair of glasses, bifocals are sometimes recommended.

EYE STRAIN

Uncorrected refractive errors or wrongly prescribed glasses may lead to symptoms which include red eyes, blurring, watering, tired eyes and headaches which may be ocular, frontal or diffuse. There is often a close relationship between eye strain and the use of the eyes for reading, driving, or an occupation which requires close visual concentration. Patients show great individual variation in the tolerance of refractive error. Some are sensitive to minor changes in their glasses while others are not bothered by gross refractive errors.

The symptoms of eye strain may also be due to muscle imbalance, poor convergence, a patient's neurotic state, or a variety of drugs; and occasionally, systemic diseases.

In presbyopic patients, the symptoms are relieved by the use of reading glasses and stronger focal light when reading.

CONTACT LENSES

Modern technological advances have made it possible to manufacture small lenses made of soft or hard plastic. These are the soft and hard contact lenses.

Optically, contact lenses function in the same way as glasses. They help to focus the image sharply on the retina.

There are several reasons why contact lenses are used. The most common one is cosmetic. The lenses are very popular with young female myopic patients who are willing to tolerate any discomfort or inconvenience in order to improve their appearance.

Contact lenses are also used by sportsmen who find that glasses fog with perspiration and by stage or television personalities who find it less attractive to wear glasses. They may be contraindicated in dusty or industrial conditions.

Soft contact lenses are sometimes used therapeutically to bandage a corneal ulcer which fails to heal or to prevent discomfort from chronic corneal epithelial disturbance.

Complications

A common complication, especially with hard lenses, is overwear. This leads to corneal oedema. The patient gives a history of having used the lenses longer than usual. He complains of pain, watering, photophobia and eyelid spasm (blepharospasm). One problem with soft lenses is infection which can lead to serious corneal ulceration. Because of complications, any contact lens wearer who complains of persistent pain or discomfort should have the cornea assessed by an ophthalmologist.

Aphakia

Aphakia is the optical condition of the eye without its lens (following cataract extraction). A strong convex (plus) lens has to be used to replace the power of the removed lens so that images can be focused on the retina. The thick cataract glasses can cause adjustment difficulty because of the optical distortion and the increased image size. The use of contact lens decreases the adjustment problems and is an advantage for those who can tolerate their use. In many countries intraocular implants are routinely inserted during surgery to overcome this problem.

Refractive surgery

Radial keratotomy is the most common surgical procedure of a variety of operations on the cornea designed to reduce refractive errors. It is used for the correction of simple myopia. Recent reports indicate that it is most effective in moderate myopia from 3-6 dioptres and in patients from 25-45 years of age. However, the operation is still controversial because the result is often unpredictable and the effectiveness may become less with time (1 or 2 years). Serious complications are uncommon. In some countries there is increasing use of this method to correct simple myopia. It is not used for high myopia.

11

OPHTHALMIC DRUGS

COMMON OCULAR DRUGS

Local eyedrops are useful for diseases affecting the anterior part of the eye. Ointments may be used instead of eyedrops. In general eyedrops are preferred as they will not blur vision and can deliver the drugs in higher concentration. Conditions affecting the back of the eye will require either subconjunctival or retrobulbar injections, or systemic therapy.

THERAPEUTIC DRUGS

These drugs are usually dispensed as eyedrops, but may be used as eye ointments.

Anti-infection eyedrops

• Antibacterial eyedrops

The commonly used antibiotic eyedrops are those which are seldom used systemically and have a broad spectrum of action. They are Chloramphenicol, Neomycin, Soframycin, Gentamicin and Polymyxin. Tetracycline or sulphur derivatives are particularly useful in the treatment of trachoma.

• Antiviral eyedrops

Idoxuridine, Adenine Arabinoside, Acycloguanosine and Trifluorothymidine eyedrops or ointment are used for herpes simplex infection of the eye.

Glaucoma therapy

Pilocarpine and Timolol eyedrops are most commonly used in open-angle glaucoma. Their usage is sometimes supplemented with Epinephrine (Adrenaline) eyedrops. When these eyedrops do not control the intraocular pressure adequately, Acetazolamide (Diamox) taken orally may be added. Acetazolamide may also be given intravenously in acute closed-angle glaucoma.

Decongestants (and antihistamine) eyedrops

There are numerous combinations of decongestants and antihistamine eyedrops used for non-specific conjunctivitis and mild allergies, and also as a placebo for tired, irritable eyes.

Tear replacement and lubricating eyedrops

Methylcellulose, Hypromellose or polyvinyl alcohol are examples of viscous, water-soluble compounds used as ocular lubricant eyedrops in the dry eye syndrome.

Mydriatics and cycloplegic eyedrops

Mydriatric and cycloplegic eyedrops are used in uveitis to dilate the pupil and to paralyze the muscles of accommodation in order to relieve pain and to prevent adhesion of the iris to the lens (posterior synechiae). They are also used in the treatment of amblyopia and sometimes after surgery. The common eyedrops used for longer action in therapy are Atropine and Homatropine.

Steroid eyedrops

Steroids are used in treating inflammation from many conditions such as iridocyclitis and surgical trauma. Because of their many complications, some of which can lead to severe visual loss, there should be specific indications for their use.

The combination of steroids with antibiotic eyedrops is particularly dangerous, especially when used for prolonged periods. The complications from steroid drops are glaucoma, cataract and aggravation of corneal infection, especially from herpes simplex and fungus.

DIAGNOSTIC DRUGS

- Short-acting mydriatic eyedrops are used for ophthalmoscopy and retinoscopy. These include Tropicamide and Phenylephrine.

- Local anaesthetic eyedrops are used for ocular examinations to overcome blepharospasm and for tonometry. Besides their diagnostic uses, local anaesthetic eyedrops are used in the removal of corneal or conjunctival foreign bodies.

- Fluorescein is used in strip-form in the assessment of corneal injury and suspected ulceration. It is also used as an intravenous preparation for fundal fluorescein angiography.

MISUSE OF EYEDROPS

Eyedrops, when misused, can lead to a number of complications.

Steroid eyedrops

The most important and common problem is the indiscriminate use of steroid eyedrops, especially in combination with a broad spectrum antibiotic. These eyedrops may cause dangerous complications with prolonged use. The complications include:

- Glaucoma
- Cataract
- Herpes simplex and fungal infection

Contaminated eyedrops

Eyedrops which have been opened and left unused for many months can be contaminated. It is important that unused eyedrops be discarded. Many countries warn consumers to discard eyedrops one month after opening.

Systemic effects

Local eyedrops, especially Atropine and related anti-cholinergics, may lead to systemic effects especially in children and infants. Pilocarpine eyedrops, if used intensively in acute glaucoma, can also cause systemic effects. 10% Phenylephrine drops may cause serious cardio-vascular effects including tachycardia and sudden increase in blood pressure. Timolol may aggravate asthma.

Local anaesthetic eyedrops

Local anaesthetic eyedrops should never be prescribed for ocular pain as they can de-epithelialize the cornea and mask serious eye complications by relieving the pain. When local anaesthetic drops are used for diagnostic purposes it is important that the patient be told not to rub the eye immediately after application to avoid corneal abrasion.

Antibiotic eyedrops

The prolong use of antibiotic eyedrops locally sometimes cause chronic conjunctivitis.

DIAGNOSTIC EYEDROPS

Main uses	(Chemical) Names	Remarks

Ophthalmoscopy	Dilators
	(1) Tropicamide
	  0.5%-1%
	(2) Cyclopentolate
	  1%-2%
	(3) Phenylephrine
	  2.5%-10%
		Short acting
		(6 hours)

Examination (blepharospasm and tonometry)	Local anaesthetic (1) Proparacaine (2) Tetracaine	Not to be used for pain relief
Staining cornea	(1) Fluorescein	Use strips. Drops may be contaminated.

THERAPEUTIC EYEDROPS

Indication	Drug
Bacterial Infection	<ul><li>Chloramphenicol</li><li>Neomycin</li><li>Gentamycin</li><li>Framycetin</li><li>Sulphacetamide</li></ul>
Anti-viral (Herpes simplex)	<ul><li>Idoxuridine</li><li>Adenine Arabino−side</li><li>Acycloguanosine</li><li>Trifluorothymidine</li><li>Vira A</li></ul>
Glaucoma	<ul><li>Pilocarpine</li><li>Timolol</li><li>Epinephrine (Adrenaline)</li></ul>
Chronic non−specific conjunctivitis	Decongestants (antihistamines) Numerous:<ul><li>Phenylephrine (neosynephrine)</li><li>Naphazoline</li><li>Antazoline</li><li>Zinc Sulphate</li></ul>
Dry eye	Artifical tears<ul><li>Methylcellulose</li><li>Polyvinyl alcohol</li><li>Hypromellose</li></ul>
Iridocyclitis and after surgery	Mydriatics (dilators)<ul><li>Atropine</li><li>Homatropine</li><li>Tropicamide</li></ul>
Inflammation Iridocyclitis and after surgery	Numerous steroids:<ul><li>Hydrocortisone</li><li>Prednisolone</li><li>Dexamethasone</li></ul>

Strength	Dosage	Remarks
	Use frequently 3−4 hourly but avoid prolonged therapy	Toxic to cornea
1%−4% 0.25%−0.5% 1%−2%		Constricts pupil No effects on pupil Dilates pupil
		Often used as placebo
	Apply at least every 3 hours	
0.5% − 1% 2% − 5% 0.5% − 1%		Long−acting 1 week action 2 day action 4 hours
0.1% 0.5% 0.1%		Serious complications include: • Glaucoma • Cataract • Aggravate Herpes Simplex

INDEX

Figures in bold refer to illustrations

Figures in bold refer to illustrations

Figures in bold refer to illustrations

Figures in bold refer to illustrations